I0428081

Dr. Susan's Healthy Living
drsusanshealthyliving.com

Facebook.com/DrSusanRichards
drsusanshealthyliving@gmail.com
(650) 561-9978

Mention of specific companies or products in this book does not suggest endorsement by the author or publisher. Internet addresses and telephone numbers for resources provided in this book were accurate at the time it went to press.

ISBN 978-1511993180

Note

The information in this book is meant to complement the advice and guidance of your physician, not replace it. It is very important that any person who has medical problems be evaluated by a physician. If you are under the care of a physician, you should discuss any major changes in your regimen with him or her. Because this is a book and not a medical consultation, keep in mind that the information presented here may not apply in your particular case. In view of individual medical requirements, new research, and government regulations, it is the responsibility of the reader to validate health practices and treatments with a physician or health service.

Table of Contents

Introduction

Dear Friend,

I know that you are reading this book because you are looking for positive and effective solutions for irregular and heavy menstruation. I have written this book just for you, to share with you the all natural treatment program that I have developed and successfully treated thousands of my patients.

Irregular menstrual flow affects millions of women at different times in their lives, especially in the menopause transition (premenopause) but also during women's active reproductive years. Abnormal bleeding or spotting can even occur in the menopause when changes in the lining of the uterus occur due to cancer or hyperplasia (abnormal growth of the uterine lining) or other causes. Common causes include premenopause, endometrial hyperplasia, uterine cancer, fibroid tumors and endometriosis, although other conditions like thyroid disease, Cushing's disease and cervical polyps may also cause heavy bleeding.

Heavy menstrual bleeding can cause significant symptoms and affect the ability of many women to handle their day-to-day life in an optimal way. Often the medical problems that cause irregular and heavy bleeding can be persistent and even recurrent. Each time this occurs, stronger and more powerful medical treatments may be needed to stop the process. Treatments normally include the use of medications, hormones, and surgical procedures, even to the point of a hysterectomy.

These therapies are important and can even be lifesaving in some cases, they can often be avoided if the underlying causes of the health problems are treated with the effective, all-natural therapies that I have been sharing with my patients. Each year approximately 650, 000 women in the country undergo hysterectomies, many due heavy menstrual bleeding. While some women clearly need this procedure because of life-threatening problems such as cancer, a large percentage could avoid surgery if the underlying causes of the problems were treated.

In many cases, the factors that put women at risk originate in their lifestyles. Our bodies have an amazing ability to heal if we treat them well.

I have found through my years of practice that many women can prevent, or at least minimize, irregular and heavy menstruation through powerful alternative therapies.

In this book, I share with you the very effective and successful all natural treatment program that I developed for my patients. Thousands of women in my clinical practice have found relief from irregular and heavy menstruation with my program. I have worked closely with my patients and have developed a powerful healing program based on both a deep knowledge of the medical research and the research on alternative therapies as well as my own vast clinical experience.

In my book, I discuss the causes and symptoms of this health condition as well as how best to diagnose irregular and heavy menstruation medically. I also provide you with a very useful self-evaluation workbook to help you assess your condition, risk factors and track your progress.

I have counseled my patients as to the most effective diet, nutritional supplements, stress management and exercise routines to control and heal from this issue. I have developed recipes, meal plans, and menus as well as meditations, stress reduction therapies and even a powerful and enjoyable stretching program. I also share this extremely valuable and beneficial information with you in this book. Finally, I discuss the medical options including hormonal, drug and surgical therapies, their pros and cons. Many of my patients have been able to avoid using uncomfortable drugs and, even, hysterectomy with my program.

My program and information have been greatly beneficial to many thousands of patients and I hope that you find it very useful, as well.

How to Use This Self-Help Book

This irregular menstrual flow self-help program provides very important information for all women suffering from these problems. I have written the program so that each woman reading this book can select from a wide variety of self-help treatment options. To this end, I have included many self-help techniques. A treatment plan based on only one method that purports to be the only treatment for heavy menstrual bleeding will work for only a small percentage of women. In my medical practice, I have found that results are much better if I completely individualize each patient's treatment program. By overlapping treatments from various disciplines, most women find combinations that work for them. You will be able to find a combination that works for you, too.

This program is set up so that you can develop your own treatment plan. All the methods you need are contained in this book, including information on diet and nutrition as well as beneficial vitamins, minerals, and herbs. Nutritional supplementation is a very important part of an optimal health program for any woman with heavy menstrual bleeding. I have also included suggestions for stress-reduction techniques, exercises for fitness and flexibility, acupressure massage, and stretches that are specifically helpful for symptoms arising from irregular and heavy menstruation.

First, read through the book to familiarize yourself with the material. The Workbook (Chapter 3) can help you evaluate your symptoms, and the Summary Treatment Chart for Irregular Menstruation (in Chapter 4) directs you to the treatments appropriate for your particular set of problems. These tools are quick and easy to use and will save you countless hours of work on your own. You can discover simply and easily what will work: Try all the therapies listed under your symptoms and you will probably find that some make you feel better than others. On a regular basis, do those techniques that provide relief for your symptoms. Establish a regimen that works for you and use it every day.

This program is practical and easy to follow. It can be used by itself or in conjunction with a medical program. And best of all, it works. The feeling of wellness that can be yours with a self-help program will radiate and touch your whole life. You will have more time and energy to enjoy your work, family, and other pleasures. Most of my patients tell me that their lives have been positively transformed by following these beneficial self-help techniques.

Love,

Dr. Susan

Part I:
Learning About the Problem

1

What Is Irregular Menstruation?

Irregular and heavy menstrual bleeding is a relatively common issue in women. This condition is usually called "menorrhagia" by your physician and refers to blood loss that occurs either in a rapid, heavy menstrual flow or in a more moderate flow over an unusually long period of time. Blood loss is not always limited to the duration of the menstrual cycle; some women spot between periods. Spotting also occasionally happens at mid-cycle as an accompaniment to "mittelschmerz," or the slight pain that occurs at ovulation.

Heavy, profuse menstrual bleeding can be an uncomfortable experience. Some women need to use double pads or a pad and a tampon and must change them frequently, as often as every hour or two in severe cases. Many times, even frequent changes of pads and tampons do not soak up all the blood loss. Excessive menstrual flow can stain underwear and clothing, often at the most inopportune times, which can obviously be unpleasant and embarrassing. Profuse menstrual flow can also be accompanied by large blood clots, which can be painful to pass and may leave a woman feeling weak, fatigued, and literally drained of energy for a day or two each month. If this process is allowed to go untreated, the excessive blood loss over time can lead to anemia.

The Normal Menstrual Cycle

Let us look at the normal menstrual cycle and see how it functions. Once you understand the workings of a normal cycle, it will be much easier for you to understand the changes that can occur to disrupt this normal pattern and cause excessive menstrual bleeding.

First, it's important to understand why menstruation occurs. Menstruation refers to the shedding of the uterine lining, or endometrium. Each month the uterus prepares a thick, blood-rich cushion to nourish and house a fertilized egg. If conception occurs, the endometrium becomes the placenta. If pregnancy doesn't occur, the egg doesn't implant in the uterus and the body doesn't need the extra buildup of uterine lining. The uterus cleanses itself by releasing the extra blood and tissue so that the buildup can recur the following month.

The mechanism that regulates the buildup and shedding of the uterine lining is controlled by fluctuations in hormonal levels, specifically the female hormones estrogen and progesterone. (Fluctuations in these two hormones are based on a feedback system in which several of the endocrine glands secrete chemicals called hormones.) Hormones enter the bloodstream where they circulate to a target gland. The hormone acts as a messenger, instructing the target gland to make its own hormone. In other cases, the hormone can trigger chemical reactions in other parts of the body.

Let's look at the way this feedback system operates in the menstrual cycle. Three glands are directly involved in turning menstruation on and off: the hypothalamus, the pituitary, and the ovaries. Other glands, such as the adrenals and thyroid, are also necessary for healthy menstrual function.

The initial trigger for the menstrual cycle comes from hormones produced in the hypothalamus, a walnut-sized collection of highly specialized brain cells located above the pituitary. The hypothalamus regulates many basic bodily functions besides the production of female sex hormones, including temperature control, sleep patterns, thirst, and hunger. The hypothalamus is very sensitive to stresses such as emotional problems and infections. Severe stresses can affect the ability of the hypothalamus to pass signals to the pituitary and from there to the other endocrine glands. This can cause imbalances in the menstrual cycle.

The pituitary, located at the base of the brain, stimulates all the glands of the body and provides the next mechanism in regulating the menstrual cycle. To communicate with the pituitary, the hypothalamus releases messengers into the bloodstream called FSH-RF (follicle-stimulating horm-one — releasing factor) and LH-RF (luteinizing hormone — releasing factor).

When these messages from the hypothalamus are received, the pituitary begins to produce its own hormones. It triggers the menstrual cycle and ovulation by secreting FSH (follicle-stimulating hormone) and LH (luteinizing hormone). It also triggers adrenal function through the production of ACTH (adrenocorticotrophic hormone) and thyroid function through TSH (thyroid-stimulating hormone).

Once FSH and LH are released into the bloodstream, their destinations are the ovaries, the female reproductive organ. The ovaries are two small, almond-shaped glands located in a woman's pelvis. The ovaries hold all the eggs a woman will ever have, in an inactive form called follicles. At birth, each female has about 1 million follicles. By puberty, the number of eggs has been reduced to 300,000 to 400,000. The eggs decrease in number throughout a woman's life, until menopause, at which time the follicles have atrophied and lost their ability to produce estrogen. Without sufficient estrogen, menstruation ceases.

Each month, FSH and LH from the pituitary cause the follicles to ripen and release an egg for possible fertilization. (Usually only one ovary is stimulated in a cycle.) In doing so, the follicles begin to produce the hormones estrogen and progesterone. Estrogen reaches its peak during the first half of the cycle, while progesterone output occurs after midcycle when ovulation has occurred. Ovulation refers to the production of a mature egg cell, which travels down the fallopian tube to the uterus. Fertilization normally occurs in the fallopian tube. Besides preparing the egg for fertilization, estrogen and progesterone stimulate the lining of the uterus.

During the first two weeks following menstruation, estrogen causes the uterine lining to gradually rebuild itself. The glands of the endometrium begin to grow long and the lining thickens through an increase in the number of blood vessels as well as the production of a mesh of fibers that interconnect throughout the lining. By midcycle, the lining of the uterus has increased three times in thickness and has a greatly increased blood supply.

After midcycle, usually around day 14, ovulation occurs and the egg is picked up by a fallopian tube for the journey to the uterus. The follicle that produced the egg for that month (or Graafian follicle) is further stimulated after midcycle by LH and changes into the yellow body, or corpus luteum. The corpus luteum secretes progesterone — the second ovarian hormone of the menstrual cycle - which causes a coiling of the blood vessels of the uterine lining. The uterine lining becomes swollen and tortuous and secretes a thick mucous.

If the egg is fertilized, it will implant on the uterine wall and the corpus luteum will continue to secrete progesterone. If no fertilization occurs, the corpus luteum begins to deteriorate and the progesterone levels decrease. The lining of the uterus starts to break down and menstruation begins. Normal menstruation lasts three to five days. However, bleeding patterns can vary and be as short as two days or as long as seven days for some women.

What Causes Irregular Menstruation?

The normal menstrual cycle should function smoothly and without complications during a woman's active reproductive years — beginning in her early teens to about age fifty. Yet there are a variety of health and environmental issues that can disrupt a normal menstrual pattern and cause irregular and excessive bleeding. One very common problem is dysfunctional uterine bleeding. It is primarily caused by lack of ovulation which results in a lack of progesterone production during the second half of the menstrual cycle. This usually occurs frequently at either end of the reproductive cycle — in puberty and during perimenopause (the time of transition into menopause).

During adolescence, a woman's estrogen levels are gradually increasing. While her menstrual cycle is in the process of establishing itself on a mature adult basis, ovulation is often infrequent or sporadic. As a result, an adolescent may have periods that are heavier, longer, or closer together than those of adult women. Menstrual cycles that occur without ovulation are called anovulatory cycles. After a few years of menstruation, this pattern of heavy menstrual bleeding tends to self-correct as ovulation begins to occur on a regular basis.

At the other end of the spectrum, as women approach menopause, their follicles gradually atrophy and diminish in number. This transition period can last as long as four to five years. As their follicles lose the ability to produce estrogen and progesterone, perimenopausal women begin to ovulate less frequently. For many women, the transitions into menopause can be uncomfortable and difficult experiences.

As the hormonal output becomes unstable during a woman's mid to late forties, irregular and heavy bleeding may occur. The menstrual cycle often shortens, with periods coming closer together. Bleeding may become heavier and last longer. A one-week to ten-day menstrual period is fairly common. Some patients tell me that their cycles are unpredictable, sometimes coming twice a month, and in some extreme cases lasting as long as 60 or more days. This blood loss can be dangerous because it can lead to anemia if not treated. As with most menstrual problems that women encounter while entering adolescence, unpredictable cycles eventually correct themselves. When menopause approaches, the periods occur at longer intervals and the flow becomes light and scanty until menstruation finally ceases.

If the bleeding is found to be due only to the hormonal instability that occurs prior to menopause, the symptoms may recur throughout the transition into menopause. Women are most likely to have a hysterectomy performed during this time. Over 650,000 hysterectomies are done each year in the United States. Interestingly enough, only 10 to 12 percent are done for life-threatening reasons, such as cancer.

During my practice, I have found that many cases of irregular and heavy menstrual bleeding can be treated in a conservative, nonsurgical fashion by employing supportive therapy such as nutrition and stress management and, as necessary, hormonal therapy. If a woman with heavy menstrual bleeding due to hormonal instability can get through the transition period and avoid a hysterectomy, the problem will often self-correct with menopause, and the woman will have avoided major surgery. Of course, this is not always possible, and there are cases of serious profuse bleeding in which a hysterectomy may be the only sensible and correct solution.

You should be aware that menstrual bleeding is affected by many environmental factors. For example, cigarette smoking and excessive alcohol intake can worsen menstrual bleeding. Alcohol, if used in excess, is toxic to the liver. The liver is responsible for the breakdown of the estrogen so that it can be excreted from the body. If the liver is not functioning properly, the circulating levels of estrogen may be too high and thus worsen the bleeding problem.

Stress of all kinds can worsen menstrual bleeding. The menstrual cycle is ultimately dependent on the smooth functioning of the endocrine glands. As mentioned earlier, the normal functioning of the hypothalamus in the brain is strongly affected by major stresses of any kind. Traumas such as divorce, death of a loved one, job changes, moving to a new home, or even taking a major trip can impact the menstrual cycle of a susceptible woman. Helpful techniques to deal with stress are included in the self-help section of this book.

Regular menstrual cycles depend not only on emotional health but also on good nutritional habits. Women who are grossly overweight produce higher levels of estrogen and are at greater risk of anovulatory cycles and heavy menstrual bleeding. For these women, a low-fat, low-sugar diet is mandatory. An optimal diet will contain plenty of high-nutrient foods, such as whole grains, beans, peas, fresh fruits and vegetables, raw seeds and nuts, and fish (for women who eat meat as a main form of protein). Women who eat a nutrient-poor diet are also at high risk of heavy menstrual bleeding because they lack the nutrients to regulate normal blood flow.

Medical studies have shown that deficiencies of vitamin A, vitamin C, iron, and bioflavonoids can worsen or even cause heavy, irregular menstrual bleeding. These nutrients should be included in both the diets and supplement programs of women with heavy bleeding. The self-help section of this book provides detailed information on foods, vitamins, minerals, and herbs that help to control heavy menstrual flow.

While many cases of irregular and heavy menstrual flow are due to hormonal imbalances, other medical problems can also cause bleeding. One of the most common is fibroid tumors. Fibroids, also called myomas, are benign growths of muscle and connective tissue, usually found in the wall of the uterus. They are a common condition affecting 40 percent of all American women. For most women, fibroids do not create a problem if their tumors are small and don't cause any symptoms. However, for some women in their thirties and forties, fibroids can become a real problem. In these women, the fibroids either grow to be so large or become so numerous that they put pressure on the bowel or bladder wall, causing discomfort, frequent urination, and changes in bowel habits. At times, the fibroids grow to be so large that a woman feels them in her uterus through the abdominal wall, and she can appear to be four to five months pregnant. Sometimes fibroids outgrow their blood supply, causing much discomfort. Fibroids can also cause heavy menstrual bleeding, which can lead to anemia.

Fibroids are one of the most common causes of hysterectomies in women. Like the heavy menstrual bleeding seen in perimenopausal women, fibroids are stimulated by unopposed high levels of estrogen. For this reason, women with fibroids should avoid birth control pills, estrogen replacement therapy after menopause, alcohol, high-fat diets, and excessive life stresses, since these factors can stimulate high levels of estrogen. Vitamin E, vitamin B complex, and herbs that have low levels of progesterone or help optimize liver function may be helpful in treating fibroids. Information about diet and supplements that are helpful for fibroids can be found in the self-help section of this book.

Because fibroids are stimulated by estrogen, they tend to shrink in size after menopause. If a woman can avoid having a hysterectomy during the transition period, she may have no further problems once menstruation ends. For women whose symptoms require a surgical treatment for their fibroids, several options are available. A young woman who wishes to have children at a later date may elect to have a myomectomy, a procedure that removes only the fibroids. This may relieve the pain and bleeding, but further surgery may be needed later if the fibroids continue to grow. Women who are past their childbearing years and have uncomfortable bowel or bladder symptoms or severe bleeding may require a hysterectomy. However, unless the fibroids actually cause symptoms or show signs of malignancy (which is very rare), they do not need to be removed. In my opinion, many gynecologists recommend hysterectomies that are unnecessary.

Other abnormal uterine growths are stimulated by excessive levels of estrogen and can cause profuse bleeding as the initial symptom. Overgrowth of the uterine lining (endometrial hyperplasia) uterine endometrial polyps and uterine (endometrial) cancer tend to be seen in older women or those who are in transition into menopause. Risk factors associated with cancerous or precancerous growths of the uterus include obesity, hypertension, diabetes mellitus, childlessness, and a history of breast cancer. Using unopposed estrogen without progesterone for postmenopausal hormonal replacement therapy increases a woman's risk of developing uterine cancer fivefold. Dietary and stress factors also increase the risk of excessive estrogen levels. Cancer of the uterus and precancerous lesions are linked to excessive bleeding before, during, or after menstruation, as well as postmenopausal bleeding and spotting. Bleeding in a postmenopausal woman should be evaluated carefully to find the possible cause.

Another cause of excessive bleeding is endometriosis, a condition in which the cells of the lining of the uterus (or endometrium) break away and grow outside the uterine cavity, implanting themselves in the pelvis. These implants can appear in a bewildering variety of locations throughout the pelvis including the ovaries, the ligaments of the uterus, the cervix, appendix, bowel and bladder. Occasionally, these cells can even invade distant structures such as a lung or armpit. Like the regular lining of the uterus, endometrial implants respond to hormonal stimulation and can cause bleeding in the pelvic cavity. Unlike normal menstrual bleeding, implant bleeding cannot leave the body through the vaginal opening during menstruation. Instead, blood from the endometrial implants remains trapped in the pelvis, causing inflammation, cysts, scar tissue, and other structural damage to the tissues and organs in this area.

Abnormal bleeding, including premenstrual spotting and excessive menstrual flow, occurs in approximately one third of women with endometriosis and may be due to lack of ovulation. In anovulatory cycles, progesterone is not produced. Progesterone has an important effect on the uterine lining during the normal menstrual cycle and helps to limit the amount of blood flow. Bleeding can be excessive without it and if excessive bleeding or spotting happens too frequently, iron-deficiency anemia may occur.

Additional causes of abnormal or excessive bleeding include cervical erosions or polyps, hypothyroidism, Cushing's disease (a disease of the adrenal glands), pituitary tumors, blood clotting abnormalities, the use of an IUD, and even complications from pregnancy. The presence of an IUD can also cause excessive menstrual bleeding.

Diagnosis of Irregular Menstruation

With so many health issues linked to irregular and heavy menstrual flow, the importance of a thorough diagnostic evaluation can't be overestimated. As mentioned earlier, heavy flow is usually due to hormonal imbalance, although it can also be the result of uterine fibroids, polyps, or even uterine or cervical cancer. Though the likelihood is small, these problems must be diagnosed early for the best prognosis.

Women with bleeding problems need to have a careful medical history taken and a physical examination. A pelvic exam can detect obvious causes of bleeding such as cervical erosion or polyps. A complete blood count should be done to check for anemia, as well as blood clotting abnormalities, and hypothyroidism which also cause heavy menstruation. A PAP smear will help rule out cervical cancer and can detect some cases of endometrial cancer. The most accurate diagnostic test for heavy bleeding is an endometrial biopsy. This can be done in your doctor's office and involves the removal of a small sample of the uterine lining by means of a thin pipette curette. The collected cells are examined under a microscope for any abnormalities that suggest hyperplasia or cancer.

Occasionally, a more extensive procedure called a dilation and curettage (D&C) may be performed if the patient is experiencing particularly heavy blood loss, or if polyps are suspected. The D&C requires anesthesia and removes samples of the uterine lining using a scraping or suction technique. In addition to its diagnostic use, the D&C also effectively stops the bleeding, at least temporarily.

Your physician may also recommend an imaging technique called an ultrasound which can visualize the size and shape of any pelvic masses. Ultrasound can also be used to assess the thickness of the uterine lining in the diagnosis of hyperplasia. Once the cause of the bleeding is accurately pinpointed, the appropriate treatment can be prescribed.

Part II:
Evaluating Your Symptoms

2

The Irregular Menstruation Workbook

This workbook section will help you evaluate your symptoms as well as the factors that contribute to your risk of developing irregular and heavy menstrual bleeding. It is important to be aware of your risk factors since these problems can recur throughout your reproductive years. Luckily, you can eliminate many risk factors by modifying your lifestyle habits.

If you take the time to fill out the evaluation sheets, you will find it easier to recognize your weak areas; then you can put together your own treatment program from the following chapters for the best relief and prevention of irregular and heavy menstrual bleeding.

First, fill out the checklist to evaluate your symptoms. Then, carefully assess your responses for the risk factors for irregular and heavy menstrual bleeding. Finally, fill out the lifestyle habit evaluations related to eating and exercise. These will help you assess specific areas of your life to see which of your habit patterns are contributing to your symptoms. This evaluation will also show you if you are at risk for irregular and heavy menstrual bleeding. Working with the preventive health-care techniques in the rest of the book can help improve your health and lessen your risks.

When you have completed the evaluations, you will be ready to go on to the next chapter and begin your treatment program.

Risk Factors for Irregular Menstruation

You are at higher risk of irregular and heavy menstrual bleeding if you have any of the risk factors listed below. Be sure to follow the nutritional and other self-help techniques for uterine health. Get regular Pap smears. See your doctor if you have any abnormal vaginal bleeding after menopause because this bleeding can be a sign of uterine cancer.

	Yes	No
Lack of ovulation	____	____
Perimenopausal woman	____	____
(in transition into menopause)	____	____
Fibroid tumors	____	____
Thyroid disease	____	____
Blood coagulation problem	____	____
Uterine polyps	____	____
Menopausal woman using estrogen replacement therapy without progesterone	____	____
Obesity	____	____
Early menstruation	____	____
Childlessness	____	____
High blood pressure	____	____
Lack of iodine	____	____
Lack of iron	____	____
Lack of vitamin A	____	____
Lack of vitamin C	____	____
Lack of bioflavonoids	____	____

Lifestyle Habits for Irregular Menstruation

Eating Habits

Check the number of times you eat the following foods: Foods in shaded area are "high-stress" foods.

Foods That Increase Symptoms

Foods	Never	1x a Month	1x a Week	>1x a Week
Coffee				
Cow's milk				
Cow's cheese				
Butter				
Chocolate				
Sugar				
Alcohol				
Wheat bread				
Wheat noodles				
Wheat-based flour				
Pastries				
Added salt				
Bouillon				
Commercial salad dressing				
Catsup				
Black tea				
Soft drinks				
Hot dogs				
Ham				
Bacon				
Beef				
Lamb				
Pork				

Foods That Decrease Symptoms

Foods	Never	1x a Month	1x a Week	>1x a Week
Avocado				
Green Beans				
Beets				
Broccoli				
Brussels sprouts				
Cabbage				
Carrots				
Celery				
Collard greens				
Cucumbers				
Eggplant				
Garlic				
Horseradish				
Kale				
Legumes				
Lettuce				
Mustard greens				
Okra				
Onions				
Parsnips				
Peas				
Potatoes				
Radishes				
Rutabagas				
Spinach				
Squash				
Sweet potatoes				
Tomatoes				
Turnips				
Turnip greens				
Yams				
Brown rice				
Millet				
Barley				
Oatmeal				
Buckwheat				
Rye				
Raw flaxseeds				
Corn				

Raw sesame seeds				
Raw sunflower seeds				
Raw almonds				
Raw filberts				
Raw pecans				
Raw pumpkin seeds				
Raw walnuts				
Apples				
Bananas				
Berries				
Pears				
Seasonal fruits				
Corn oil				
Flax oil				
Olive oil				
Sesame oil				
Safflower oil				
Eggs				
Poultry				
Fish				

Key to Eating Habits

Irregular menstrual bleeding tendencies are greatly affected by the quality of your nutritional habits: The production of healthy red blood cells and the ability to regulate menstrual flow depend on an abundance of nutrients such as iron, vitamin B12, folic acid, vitamin B6, vitamin E, bioflavonoids, and vitamin C, as well as other essential nutrients.

All foods on the preceding list in the shaded area are high-stress foods that can worsen your menstrual bleeding problems. If you eat large numbers of these foods, or if you eat any of these foods frequently, your nutritional habits may be contributing significantly to your symptoms, and you can probably benefit greatly from the dietary guidelines in the nutritional chapters. All foods listed from avocados to fish are high-nutrient, low-stress foods. Many contain one or more of the essential nutrients needed to relieve and prevent irregular and heavy menstrual bleeding.

Key to Exercise Habits

Many women with irregular and heavy menstrual bleeding tend to have major problems with fatigue as well as lack of physical endurance and stamina. Even women who have been used to an active and vigorous exercise regimen may feel that any physical activity at all is just too difficult and may decide to stop exercising completely. This can have negative physiological effects on the body and increase the symptoms. While vigorous exercise may indeed exhaust a woman suffering from anemia, gentle and moderate exercise can provide the benefits of oxygenation and improved blood circulation. Select one or two of the less strenuous exercises given in the checklist and do them two to three times per week. Chapters 9 and 10 describe gentle exercise routines that you may find pleasant and easy to do.

Exercise Habits

Check the number of times you do each of the following activities:

Activity	Never	Once a Month	Once a Week	Twice a Week +
Walking				
Swimming				
Bicycling				
Stretching				
Stretches				
Golf				
Weight lifting (low stress)				
T'ai chi				
Ballroom dancing				

Key to Areas of Tension

This evaluation should help you become aware of how irregular menstrual flow can affect muscle tension in your body. Each woman has her own particular area where she localizes muscle tension. Irregular and heavy menstruation reduces the amount of oxygen available to all the tissues of the body. There is a resultant accumulation of carbon dioxide and lactic acid. These waste products cause muscle contraction, as well as an increase in your level of fatigue and a decrease in your sense of vitality.

Try to remain aware of the areas in your body where you store tension. When you feel tension building up in them, do the stretches and stress-reduction exercises described in this book. They will help to reduce the tension significantly.

Areas of Tension

Check the places where tension most commonly localizes in your body:

Location	Never	Seldom	Often	Always
Shoulder				
Neck and throat				
Grinding teeth				
Lower back				
Headache				
Eyestrain				
Arms				
Stomach muscles				

Key to Stress Symptoms

Women with irregular menstrual bleeding may notice changes in their emotional state because of the fatigue and low energy that accompany these conditions. As a result of fatigue, feelings of hopelessness and depression may occur. If you have any of these symptoms, look at the many self-help treatment options described in this book. Try several of them and see which ones make you feel the best.

Stress Symptoms

Check the degree to which you are affected by the following symptoms:

Symptom	Never	Mildly	Moderately	Severely
Dizziness				
Decreased mental acuity				
Feeling constantly stressed				
Tension				
Mood swings				
Fatigue				
Depression				
Hopelessness				
Low self-esteem				

Part III:
Finding the Solution

3

Self-Help Program - A Summary Treatment Chart

Now that you have read about the symptoms and causes of irregular menstrual bleeding, you are ready to put together your own self-help treatment program. I have included in this part of the book many treatment methods that I have found to be helpful with my patients. These treatment options include dietary and nutritional supplement programs as well as programs for stress management, exercise, acupressure, and stretches. Each of the following chapters presents specific information and techniques to help relieve and prevent irregular and heavy menstrual bleeding.

The program is set up so that you can individualize a treatment plan for yourself. This chapter contains a summary chart that will help you put your own program together. The chart lists all the treatments in this book that you can use for irregular and heavy menstrual bleeding.

There are two ways that you might use the summary chart. First, you can identify your problem in the chart and turn directly to the treatments for the problem. I recommend that when beginning a program, you try all the therapies listed for your problem. You will probably find that some techniques make you feel better than others. Establish the regimen that works for you and practice it on a regular basis. Alternatively, you can read straight through the rest of the book to get a general overview of the various treatment techniques. Find the treatments that you are interested in trying; then use the treatment chart for an overview and quick spot work.

Either way of working with the book can bring you tremendous benefits. The most important thing is to follow your program on a regular basis.

This will enable you to see improvement in your health and vitality very quickly-many women begin to feel better within a month or two.

Summary Treatment Chart for Irregular Menstruation

Medication	Progestins Natural progesterone Nonsteroidal anti-inflammatory drugs (Motrin, Anaprox, etc.)
Vitamins and Minerals	Heavy bleeding formula with emphasis on vitamin A, vitamin C, bioflavonoids, and iron
Herbs	Flax oil and flax meal, soy isoflavones, shepherd's purse, golden seal, silymarin, curcumin, grape skins, cherry, bilberry, huckleberry
Nutrition	Irregular and Heavy Menstruation self-help diet
Stress Reduction	Stress reduction exercises 1, 3, 5, 7
Exercise	Exercises 1, 2, 3
Stretches	Stretches 1, 2, 3, 4
Acupressure	Acupressure exercises 1, 2, 3, 4, 5

4

Vitamins, Minerals & Herbs

The use of vitamins, minerals, and herbs is extremely important for both the treatment and the prevention of irregular and heavy menstrual bleeding. In order to be symptom-free, you must have an optimal intake of the nutrients necessary for the growth and production of red blood cells and for the regulation of bleeding. I have found that my patients heal most effectively when they combine a nutrient-rich diet with the right mix of supplements. Though nothing can replace a healthful diet, most women have difficulty using diet alone to increase their nutrient intake to the levels needed for optimal healing. The use of supplements can help correct this deficiency so you can heal as rapidly and completely as possible.

As you read this chapter, you will learn about the beneficial effects that nutrition can have on fatigue, depression, low energy, poor digestion, and other symptoms of irregular and heavy menstrual bleeding. In fact, poor or inadequate nutrition may play a major role in causing these problems or contribute greatly to their onset.

This chapter is divided into three sections. The first discusses the role of vitamins and minerals in the body, along with their major food sources. The next section tells which herbs are helpful for irregular and heavy menstrual bleeding and why they are effective. The third section gives specific recommendations on how to use these supplements for irregular and heavy menstruation.

Toward the end of the chapter I have included several charts listing major food sources of each essential nutrient. The importance of nutrition in regulating irregular and heavy menstrual bleeding is supported by numerous medical studies done at university centers and hospitals; a bibliography is included at the end of this chapter for those wanting more technical information.

Vitamins and Minerals for Irregular Menstruation

Vitamin A: Vitamin A is necessary for the normal growth and support of the eyes, skin, and mucous membranes and healthy immune function. Deficiency of vitamin A results in impaired immune function; rough, scaly skin; and night blindness. It is also needed for the healthy production of red blood cells. In an interesting study of middle-aged men on a diet deficient in vitamin A, it was found that the hemoglobin count started to decline even before a change in night vision or a measurable deficiency in the vitamin A levels was noted. Vitamin A also plays a significant role in the prevention of heavy menstrual bleeding. In a study of 71 women with excessive bleeding, the women were found to have significantly lower blood levels of vitamin A than the normal population. Almost 90 percent of the women studied returned to a normal bleeding pattern after two weeks of vitamin A treatment.

There are two types of vitamin A. Vitamin A from animal sources usually comes from fish liver and is oil soluble. This type of vitamin A can be toxic if taken in too large a dose (i.e., greater than 25,000 international units [I.U.] per day, if taken for more than a few months). In contrast, beta carotene, the precursor of vitamin A found in plants, is water soluble and is not toxic in large amounts. A single sweet potato or cup of carrot juice contains more than 20,000 I.U. of beta carotene.

Vitamin B Complex: The vitamin B complex consists of eleven factors that work together to perform many important biochemical functions in the body. These functions include stabilization of brain chemistry, glucose metabolism, and the inactivation of estrogen by the liver. Since heavy menstrual bleeding can be due to excess estrogen in the body, it is important that estrogen levels are properly regulated through breakdown and disposal by the liver. Vitamin B factors are essential for healthy liver functioning.

The B-complex vitamins are also necessary for the prevention and reversal of anemia. A deficiency of vitamin B1 (thiamine), vitamin B2 (riboflavin), vitamin B5 (pantothenic acid), and vitamin B6 (pyridoxine) may cause anemia, even in people who have no deficiencies in iron, folic acid, or vitamin B12. The B-complex vitamins are commonly found in foods such as whole grains, beans and peas, and liver. These vitamins are water soluble. When a woman is under emotional stress, the B-complex vitamins are more easily lost from the body. This can worsen the fatigue and lack of vitality from which women with heavy menstrual bleeding already suffer. Dosage is 25 to 100 mg per day.

Folic Acid: Folic acid is one of the B-complex vitamins and is an important nutrient for women. It helps prevent cervical dysplasia, a condition that can be a precursor to cancer of the cervix. It is also a necessary supplement for women who use birth control pills, since oral contraceptives interfere with folic acid absorption. Deficiency of folic acid in pregnant women has been linked to neural tube defects in their babies, such as spina bifida. Folic acid plays an important role in the production of red blood cells.

A deficiency of folic acid leads to anemia that cannot be corrected by supplemental iron. With folic acid deficiency, red blood cells do not mature properly; they are large and irregularly shaped. Drugs that interfere with proper folic acid absorption include sulfa drugs and other antibiotics, phenobarbital, alcohol, and anticonvulsants used in the treatment of epilepsy. Women with folic acid deficiency anemia are prone to symptoms such as sore tongue, digestive disturbances, forgetfulness, and mental confusion. Good food sources of folic acid include oysters, salmon, whole grains, and green leafy vegetables. Dosage is 400 mg to 1 gram per day.

Vitamin B12: Vitamin B12 is a water-soluble vitamin that plays an important role in the production of red blood cells. Like folic acid deficiency, a B12 deficiency causes retardation in the growth and development of the red blood cells. Vitamin B12 is poorly absorbed from the gastrointestinal tract if the intrinsic factor, a necessary enzyme, is deficient. Since vitamin B12 is found primarily in meat, vegetarians may be at risk of developing a B12 deficiency. Symptoms of this deficiency develop slowly and may not become apparent for as long as five or six years.

A lack of B12 causes symptoms such as shooting pains, pins-and-needles or hot-and-cold sensations in the extremities, as well as numbness, stiffness, and difficulty in walking. It can also cause mental disturbances similar to psychosis, as well as memory defects and mental slowness. In order to treat B12 deficiency anemia (or pernicious anemia), the digestive tract must be bypassed and the B12 given as injections.

Vitamin C: This important anti-stress vitamin is necessary for proper adrenal function as well as for immune function. Vitamin C increases iron absorption from the non-heme iron sources such as bran, peas, seeds, nuts, and leafy green vegetables. This can help to prevent iron deficiency anemia. Vitamin C has also been tested, along with bioflavonoids, as a treatment for heavy menstrual bleeding. One study showed a reduction in bleeding in 87 percent of the women participating. Vitamin C strengthens capillaries and prevents capillary fragility, which can lead to excessive bleeding. Fruits and vegetables are excellent sources of vitamin C. Dosage is 800 to 2000 mg per day.

Soy Isoflavones: Genistein and diadzein are isoflavones found in soy with weak estrogen-like activity. They help to reduce excess estrogen levels by interfering with estrogen production and the binding of estrogen to tissues such as the breast and uterus. In fact, a study of Hawaiian women found that using soy actively reduced the risk of endometrial (uterine) cancer by 54 percent.

Bioflavonoids: Bioflavonoids have chemical activity similar to estrogen and can be used as an estrogen substitute. Clinical studies have shown that bioflavonoids help to control hot flashes and the psychological symptoms of menopause, including anxiety, irritability, and mood swings. Interestingly, bioflavonoids contain a very low potency of estrogen, much lower than that used as hormonal replacement therapy. As a result, no harmful side effects have been noted with bioflavonoid therapy.

Bioflavonoids, along with vitamin C, reduce heavy menstrual bleeding due to hormonal imbalance by strengthening the capillary walls. They have even been used to treat women who have lost multiple pregnancies due to bleeding. In nature, bioflavonoids are found in fruits, such as citrus rind and pulp, grape skins, cherries, blackberries, as well as vegetables. Dosage is 700 to 2000 mg per day.

Flaxseeds: Flaxseeds contain both omega-3 essential fatty acids and lignans which make up the cellular wall of the seeds. Both substances are weakly estrogenic and help reduce estrogen levels within the body, as well as promoting healthy ovulation. This was researched with positive results in a study at the University of Minnesota. In my medical practice I have found flaxseed oil to be an effective menstrual regulator. Use 1 to 3 tablespoons per day as an oil or butter substitute.

Vitamin E: Vitamin E can act as a weak estrogen substitute. It has been studied as a treatment for hot flashes, the psychological symptoms of menopause, and even vaginal dryness. In one study, vitamin E was found to help skew the estrogen-progesterone ratio in the body toward progesterone and is needed for normal ovulation. It is helpful for those women who have heavy menstrual bleeding due to excess estrogen. Vitamin E also protects the cells from the destructive effects of environmental pollutants that can react with the cell membrane. It increases red blood cell survival and is an important nutrient for the prevention of anemia. Vitamin E is found in wheat germ, nuts, and seeds. Dosage is 400 to 1600 IU per day.

Vitamin K: Vitamin K is an amazing nutrient that does double duty in protecting both your bones and circulation! If you bruise easily, have bleeding of your gums, heavy menstrual bleeding, osteoporosis or calcification of your arteries, you are probably vitamin K deficient. In fact, it is important to have sufficient vitamin K in your diet when following a program to combat irregular and heavy menstrual bleeding.

Great sources of this essential vitamin include my favorite greens- kale, collard, spinach, mustard greens, Swiss chard and parsley. Other excellent foods include broccoli, romaine lettuce, tomatoes, asparagus and cucumbers (with skin on). Dosage that I recommend is 100 mcg per day if you would like to take vitamin K as a supplement.

Iron: Women who suffer from heavy menstrual bleeding tend to be iron deficient. In fact, some medical studies have found that inadequate iron intake may be a cause of excessive bleeding as well as an effect of the problem. Women who suffer from heavy menstrual bleeding should have their red blood count checked to see if supplemental iron is necessary due to anemia, in addition to adopting a high-iron-content diet. Heme iron, the iron from meat sources such as liver, is much better absorbed and assimilated than non-heme iron, the iron from vegetarian sources. To be absorbed properly, non-heme iron must be taken with at least 75 milligrams of vitamin C. For more information about food combinations that are high in both iron and vitamin C, see the following two chapters on dietary planning.

Iron deficiency, often due to irregular and heavy menstruation, is the main cause of anemia in many women. Iron is an essential component of red blood cells, combining with protein and copper to make hemoglobin, the pigment of the red blood cells. Iron deficiency is common during all phases of a woman's life and is a frequent cause of fatigue and low-energy states. Good food sources of iron include liver, blackstrap molasses, beans and peas, seeds and nuts, and certain fruits and vegetables.

Copper: Copper aids in the formation of red blood cells. A deficiency of copper is associated with anemia, since copper is necessary for proper iron absorption. Copper is found in all body tissues and is present in many of the enzymes that break down and build up body tissues. The best food sources of copper include liver, whole grains, legumes, seafood, and green leafy vegetables.

Zinc: Zinc plays an important role in the body. It is a constituent of many enzymes involved both in metabolism and digestion. It is also needed for the proper growth and development of female reproductive organs and for the normal functioning of the male prostate gland. Good food sources of zinc include wheat germ, pumpkin seeds, whole grains, wheat bran, and high-protein foods. Persons who have sickle-cell anemia may be deficient in zinc. One interesting clinical study showed a decrease in the number of sickled red blood cells in patients who used zinc supplementation.

Nutrients	Importance
Vitamins	
Vitamin A	Deficiency is associated with anemia due to impaired hemoglobin synthesis as well as heavy menstrual bleeding.
Vitamin B_1 (thiamine)	Deficiency may cause megaloblastic (large-shaped cells) anemia.
Vitamin B_2 (riboflavin)	Aids in formation of red blood cells. Deficiency is associated with anemia.
Vitamin B_5 (pantothenic acid)	Aids in the reversal of anemia in cases with increased iron storage in the bone marrow.
Vitamin B_6 (pyridoxine)	Deficiency causes anemia.
Vitamin B_{12} (cyanocobalamin)	Essential for normal formation of blood cells and prevention of pernicious anemia.
Folic Acid (folacin)	Necessary for red blood cell formation.
Vitamin C	Aids in absorption of iron. Deficiency is associated with heavy menstrual bleeding.
Soy Isoflavones	Helps to reduce excess estrogen.
Bioflavonoids	Deficiency is associated with heavy menstrual bleeding.
Flaxseed Oil	Promotes healthy ovulation.
Vitamin E	Protects red blood cells from destruction. Important for sickle-cell anemia and anemia associated with cystic fibrosis and pancreatic insufficiency.
Minerals	
Copper	Aids in formation of red blood cells. Deficiency is associated with anemia.
Iron	Necessary for hemoglobin formation. Deficiency causes most frequent type of anemia.
Zinc	May be deficient in sickle-cell anemia.
Other Factors	
Hydrochloric acid	If deficient, iron absorption is impaired. May affect iron deficiency anemia.

Herbs for Irregular Menstruation

Herbs can play a helpful role in your nutritional program to relieve and prevent heavy menstrual bleeding. They should be thought of as a form of extended nutrition that can be taken as either teas or capsules. Two herbs have been traditionally used to stop excessive menstrual flow and postpartum hemorrhage: golden seal and shepherd's purse. Recent research studies have supported the traditional claims made for these herbs. Golden seal contains a chemical called berberine that calms uterine muscular tension. It has also been used to calm and soothe the digestive tract.

Shepherd's purse helps promote blood clotting and has also been used to help stop menstrual bleeding. If your bleeding is excessive or irregular, consult your physician. This needs to be evaluated carefully by your physician and, if necessary, medical therapy should be instituted. Excessive and irregular bleeding can be dangerous and should never be allowed to continue without medical help. For those women for whom the menstrual flow is normal but somewhat heavier than usual, the mild properties of herbs may be helpful for symptom relief.

Plants that contain bioflavonoids may also help stop and prevent heavy menstrual bleeding. Bioflavonoids help to strengthen capillaries and, along with vitamin C, can help prevent excessive bruising as well as bleeding. They are found in the rind and pulp of citrus fruits, hawthorn berries, bilberries, cherries, and grape skins. Other herbs help to prevent anemia by providing good sources of non-heme iron. Excellent examples are yellow dock and pau d'arco. Other plants help to relieve heavy menstrual bleeding by reducing elevated levels of estrogen in the body. Soy and red clover contain estrogen-like isoflavones which both interfere with estrogen production and block the estrogen from binding to breast and uterine tissues.

Plants that improve the detoxification and breakdown of estrogen by the liver also help to reduce excessive amounts of estrogen within the body. One such herb is tumeric, or curcumin, a traditional flavoring in Indian food.

Vitex agnus, or chasteberry, has been found to improve the estrogen-to-progesterone ratio in the body by favoring the production of progesterone during the second half of the menstrual cycle. This helps limit the amount of blood lost with menstruation. Vitex acts by promoting ovulation at mid-cycle through stimulating the production of the pituitary luteinizing hormone (LK).

Silymarin, or milk thistle, protects liver functions through its flavonoid content. These flavonoids are strong antioxidants and help protect the liver from damage.

How to Use Vitamin, Mineral & Herbal Supplements

Good dietary habits and the use of supplements are a necessary combination for women who want to make up the nutritional deficiencies that accompany heavy menstrual bleeding. In order to restore the level of nutrients necessary to produce an adequate number of red blood cells as well as healthy red blood cells, dietary intake may not be sufficient. Anemic women who suffer from heavy menstrual bleeding may need to take c and follow a healthy diet to "jump start" the system into normal functioning again. This is also true for women with heavy menstrual bleeding; supplements can help re-establish a normal hormonal profile, as well as restore the strength and integrity of the capillaries and other blood vessels so that normal bleeding patterns resume.

Vitamin, mineral, and herbal supplements, however, should never be used as an excuse to continue poor dietary habits. They should be taken with high nutrient meals to maintain optimal health. With heavy menstrual bleeding, it is important to make sure that both your diet and your supplement program provide the extra nutrients that your body needs.

Nutritional Supplements for Women with Irregular Menstruation

Good dietary habits are crucial for control of irregular and heavy menstruation symptoms. But for many women, the use of nutritional supplements is important in order to achieve high levels of the essential nutrients needed to heal irregular and heavy menstruation. On the following pages is a sample of the vitamins and minerals as well as their dosages that can be used as a foundation for your program. You can also add the other nutrients like flaxseed oil and fish oil that I have discussed in this chapter to fill out your program.

You may find it easier to implement your program if you start with one of the better quality multi-nutrient products for women that are available in health food stores and through the internet and then add the remaining essential nutrients.

Remember that all women differ somewhat in their nutritional needs. If you do take the recommended vitamin or herbal supplements, I usually advise that you start with one-fourth to one-half the dose recommended in this book and work your way up slowly to the higher dosage, if needed. You may find that you do best with slightly more or less of certain ingredients.

I recommend that patients take their supplements with meals or at least a snack. Very rarely, a woman will have a digestive reaction to supplements, such as nausea or indigestion. If this happens, stop all supplements; then resume using them, adding one at a time, until you find the offending nutrient. Eliminate from your program any nutrient to which you have a reaction. If you have any specific questions, ask a health-care professional who is knowledgeable about nutrition.

Sample Nutritional Supplementation for Irregular and Heavy Menstruation

Vitamins and Minerals	Maximum Daily Dose
Vitamin A	5000 I.U.
Beta carotene (provitamin A)	10,000 – 25,000 I.U.
Vitamin B complex	
B1 (thiamine)	25 - 100 mg
B2 (riboflavin)	25 - 100 mg
B3 (niacinamide)	25 - 100 mg
B5 (pantothenic acid)	25 - 100 mg
B6 (pyridoxine)	50 – 100 mg
B12 (cyanocobalamin)	100 – 750 mcg
Folic acid	400 – 800 mcg
Biotin	200 - 500 mcg
Choline	25 - 100 mg
Inositol	25 - 100 mg
PABA	25 - 100 mg
Vitamin C (as mineral ascorbates)	1000-2000 mg
Vitamin D	1000 I.U.
Bioflavonoids	800-2000 mg
Rutin	200 mg
Vitamin E (d-alpha tocopherol acetate)	800-1600 I.U.
Calcium	1000 - 1200 mg
Magnesium	500 - 600 mg
Potassium	100 mg
Iron	18 mg
Zinc	15 mg
Iodine	150 mcg
Manganese	5 mg
Copper	2 mg
Selenium	200 mcg
Chromium	100 – 200 mcg
Boron	3 mg

Food Sources of Iron

Grains
Bran cereal (All-Bran)
Millet, dry
Wheat germ
Pasta, whole wheat
Bran muffin
Pumpernickel bread
Oak flakes
Shredded wheat
Whole wheat bread
Rye bread
Wheat bran
Pearl barley
White rice

Legumes
Black beans
Pinto beans
Garbanzo beans
Soybeans
Kidney beans
Lima beans
Lentils
Split peas
Black-eyed peas
Green peas
Tofu

Vegetables
Brussels sprouts
Spinach
Broccoli
Sweet potatoes
Dandelion greens
Green beans
Corn
Leeks
Kale
Swiss chard
Beets
Beet greens
Mushrooms
Parsnips
Carrots
Mustard greens
Green pepper
Lettuce
Turnips
Asparagus
Collards
Cauliflower
Zucchini
Winter squash
Red cabbage

More Food Sources of Iron

Fruits	Meat, Poultry, Seafood	Nuts and Seeds
Prune juice	Calf's liver	Sesame seeds
Figs	Beef liver	Sunflower seeds
Raisins	Chicken liver	Pistachios
Prunes, dried	Oysters	Pecans
Avocado	Trout	Sesame butter
Apple juice	Clams	Almonds
Dates, dried	Scallops	Hazelnuts (filberts)
Blackberries	Sardines	Walnuts
Pineapple	Shrimp	
Grape juice	Chicken	
Apricots, fresh	Haddock	
Cantaloupe	Cod	
Strawberries	Salmon	
Cherries		

Food Sources of Vitamin A

Vegetables	Fruits	Meat, Poultry, Seafood
Carrots	Apricots	Crab
Carrot juice	Avocado	Halibut
Collard greens	Cantaloupe	Liver*—all types
Dandelion greens	Mangoes	Mackerel
Green onions	Papaya	Salmon
Kale	Peaches	Swordfish
Parsley	Persimmons	
Spinach		
Sweet potatoes		
Turnip greens		
Winter squash		

Food Sources of Vitamin B Complex (including folic acid)

Vegetables, Legumes	Meat, Poultry, Seafood
Alfalfa	Egg yolks*
Artichoke	Liver*
Asparagus	
Beets	Grains
Broccoli	Barley
Brussels sprouts	Bran
Cabbage	Brown rice
Cauliflower	Corn
Corn	Millet
Garbanzo beans	Rice bran
Green beans	Wheat
Kale	Wheat germ
Leeks	
Lentils	Sweeteners
Lima beans	Blackstrap molasses
Onions	
Peas	
Pinto beans	
Romaine lettuce	
Soybeans	

* Eggs and meat must be from range fed, organic sources fed on non-pesticide fodder.

Food Sources for Vitamin B$_{12}$

Protein
Fish
Eggs
Liver

Food Sources of Vitamin B$_6$

Grains
Brown rice
Buckwheat flour
Rice bran
Rye flour
Wheat germ
Whole wheat flour

Vegetables
Asparagus
Beet greens
Broccoli
Brussels sprouts
Cauliflower
Green peas
Leeks
Sweet potatoes

Nuts and seeds
Sunflower
Seeds

Meat, Poultry, Seafood
Seafood
Chicken
Salmon
Tuna

Food Sources of Vitamin C

Fruits
Blackberries
Black currants
Cantaloupe
Elderberries
Grapefruit
Grapefruit juice
Guavas
Kiwi fruit
Mangoes
Oranges
Orange juice
Pineapple
Raspberries
Strawberries
Tangerines

Vegetables, Legumes
Asparagus
Black-eyed peas
Broccoli
Brussels sprouts
Cabbage
Cauliflower
Collards
Green onions
Green peas
Kale
Kohlrabi
Parsley
Potatoes
Rutabaga
Sweet peppers
Sweet potatoes
Tomatoes
Turnips

Meat, Poultry, Seafood
Liver – all types
Pheasant
Quail
Salmon

Food Sources of Copper

Vegetables, Legumes
Kidney beans
Lentils
Lima beans
Okra
Split peas

Nuts and seeds
Almonds
Filberts
Pecans
Pistachios
Sesame seeds
Sunflower seeds
Walnuts

Meat, Poultry, Seafood
Liver
Cod
Haddock
Halibut
Lobster
Oysters
Pike
Shrimp

Fruits
Avocado
Dried figs
Prunes
Raisins

Sweeteners
Blackstrap molasses

Food Sources of Zinc

Grains
Barley
Brown rice
Buckwheat
Corn
Cornmeal
Millet
Oatmeal
Rice bran
Rye bread
Wheat bran
Wheat germ
Wheat berries
Whole wheat bread
Whole wheat flour

Vegetables, Legumes
Black-eyed peas
Cabbage
Carrots
Garbanzo beans
Green peas
Lentils
Lettuce
Lima beans
Onions
Soy flour
Soy meal
Soy protein

Meat, Poultry, Seafood
Chicken
Oysters

Fruits
Apples
Peaches

5

Dietary Principles for Irregular Menstruation

Good nutrition is absolutely essential for women with irregular and heavy menstrual bleeding. Medical studies have shown that poor nutritional habits can aggravate both of these problems. A diet full of high-stress foods such as fat, sugar, chocolate, alcohol, and caffeine does not provide the nutrients you need for healing and repair and can actually worsen the symptoms of bleeding. In contrast, a healthful and well-chosen diet can make a tremendous difference in preventing debilitating symptoms. Irregular and heavy menstruation can be prevented and controlled, at least in part, by proper nutrition.

A healthful diet includes foods such as fresh fruits and vegetables, whole grains, beans, seeds and nuts, high-quality vegetable oils, and small amounts of fish and poultry. These high-nutrient foods, together with appropriate supplements, are absolutely necessary to pro-mote optimal health and well-being. Proper food selection is an essential part of your self-help program. In this chapter, I provide the information you need about the best foods to prevent irregular and heavy menstrual bleeding, as well as which foods to avoid.

Foods that Help Treat or Prevent Irregular Menstruation

You should emphasize the following foods in your diet. These foods will also help the healing process proceed in the fastest and most efficient manner, since they contain the building blocks that your body needs for repair.

Whole Grains. Grains are an excellent source of iron. The best sources include whole grains such as millet, barley, rye, whole wheat, oats, and brown rice. Enriched grain products such as noodles, macaroni, and white rice provide additional sources of iron. However, grains contain non-heme iron, which unlike the iron found in meat, is poorly absorbed from the digestive tract. Its absorption rate is 5 percent. (The iron from meat and eggs is absorbed five times more efficiently.) Non-heme iron is also susceptible to blocking agents, such as the tannin found in tea and the calcium in antacids and food preservatives.

However, absorption of non-heme iron can be facilitated by taking at least 75 milligrams of vitamin C per meal. Plan meals that combine grains with high vitamin C content fruits and vegetables. At breakfast, add straw-berries to your corn flakes or oatmeal, or eat a fresh orange or grapefruit. At dinner you can eat pasta or rice with vegetables like broccoli, brussels sprouts, cauliflower, or green pepper to facilitate iron absorption.

Whole grains have many other benefits, too. They are good sources of lignan, a weakly estrogenic substance that makes up part of the cell wall of the plant. Lignans compete with the estrogen produced by our body for the binding receptor sites contained within the cells of uterine and breast tissue. Because lignans are much weaker than the estrogen made by our bodies, they reduce the tendency for heavy menstrual bleeding. Fiber (the digestible part of plant foods) that is found in whole grain also helps remove excess estrogen from the body. First the fiber binds to the estrogen in the intestines, and then the estrogen is eliminated through the bowel movements. Grains are also an excellent source of B-complex vitamins, vitamin E, and various minerals, all of which are needed for both normal levels of estrogen and the production and survival of red blood cells. Oat and rice bran are particularly useful.

I generally recommend that women use whole grains and whole grain flour instead of the refined grain products for their higher nutrient and fiber content. Many women with irregular and heavy menstrual bleeding also complain of poor digestive function. If this is true for you, I recommend emphasizing all grains except whole wheat. Wheat contains a protein called gluten, which is difficult to digest and can be highly allergenic. Wheat can increase fatigue, depression, and bloating.

A wide range of whole grain products and whole grain flours is available today, including cereals, breads, crackers, pancakes, and pasta. The following choices can be prepared and eaten in a variety of ways.

Whole Grain Cereals. Puffed millet, unsweetened granola, puffed corn, and puffed rice are available as cold breakfast cereals. Cream of rye and buckwheat groats are also good sources of iron. These products can be found in health food stores. Your best bet if you shop in a supermarket is the slow-cooking, old-fashioned Quaker Oats (the quick-cooking kind is a refined grain product and should be avoided). Health food stores offer a wider choice of iron-rich cereals.

Whole Grain Breads. Many different whole grain breads are available at health food stores. Examples include breads made of rice, sesame and millet, oatmeal, soy and potato, rye, and lima beans. Choose brands made without added sugar.

Crackers. Both rye and rice crackers are available in supermarkets. Rye flour, in particular, is a good source of iron. Crackers can be used for snacks or open-faced sandwiches. Brown rice cakes are particularly good with soy spreads, tuna salad, or fruit and nut spreads.

Pancakes. Pancakes can be made with buckwheat, rice or oat flour.

Pasta. Pasta made from buckwheat, rice, corn, and soybeans are readily available in health food and ethnic food stores.

Legumes. I recommend black beans, pinto beans, kidney beans, chickpeas, lentils, lima beans, and soybean products for women with irregular and heavy menstrual bleeding. They are high in iron, copper, and zinc. Legumes are very high in B-complex vitamins, folic acid, and vitamin B6, all necessary nutrients for treating anemia. They are also excellent sources of protein and provide all the essential amino acids when eaten with grains. (Good examples include meals such as beans and rice, or cornbread and lentil soup.) Sufficient protein intake is important for healthy red blood cell development, and legumes provide an excellent, easily utilized source. Soybeans contain isoflavones which help to reduce excessively high levels of estrogen in the body. An excess of estrogen causes the lining of the uterus to thicken. As the uterine lining sloughs away during menstruation, the result can be heavy menstrual bleeding as well as endometrial hyperplasia and even cancer. A study of Hawaiian women found that those with the highest consumption of soy beans were 54 percent less likely to develop of endometrial cancer.

As with grains, legumes are an excellent source of fiber and can help digestive function. They digest slowly and can help regulate the blood sugar level. They are an excellent food for women with diabetes or blood sugar imbalances. Some women find that gas is a problem when they eat beans. Gas can be minimized by eating beans in small amounts or by using digestive enzymes.

Vegetables. These are particularly good foods for both irregular and heavy menstrual bleeding since they are extremely high in both vitamin and mineral content. Vegetables high in vitamin A have bright and attractive colors, such as yellow, red, orange, and intense green. They include sweet potatoes, carrots, squash, peppers, kale, and lettuce, as well as many other common foods. Vitamin A is a very important nutrient for the prevention of heavy menstrual bleeding; a deficiency puts you at higher risk of cervical cancer. Vitamin A is also needed for normal red blood cell production. The type of vitamin A found in vegetables is water soluble and does not accumulate in toxic levels in the body. For this reason, vegetables high in vitamin A content can be eaten in large amounts.

Many vegetables are high in vitamin C. Vitamin C, along with bioflav-onoids; helps prevent and can actually help stop excessive bleeding. It also helps women absorb iron more efficiently when foods containing both nutrients are eaten together. Like vitamin A, it seems to protect women from developing cervical cancer. Vitamin C is also important for immune function, wound healing, and stress. Vegetables high in vitamin C include broccoli, Brussels sprouts, cauliflower, kale, parsley, peppers, peas, tomatoes, and potatoes. As you can see, there are many good vegetable sources for this nutrient.

Many vegetables contain high amounts of iron. Some of the best include beet greens, swiss chard, potatoes, mushrooms, tomatoes, spinach, Brussels sprouts, sweet potatoes, broccoli, kale, and green beans. These vegetables are also good sources of other minerals, such as calcium, magnesium, and potassium. I always recommend that women eat vegetables raw or steamed to preserve the nutrient value. Be careful not to boil or overcook, because important vitamins and minerals can be lost in the cooking process.

Fruits. Fruits provide a wide range of vitamins and minerals. Fruits are a terrific source of vitamins A and C, both of which help prevent and relieve heavy menstrual bleeding. Most whole fruits contain some vitamin C, with berries, oranges, grapefruits, and melons being excellent sources of this essential nutrient. Fruits that are orange and yellow in color, such as apricots, tangerines, papayas, and persimmons, are excellent sources of vitamin A.

Fresh and dried fruits are an excellent dietary substitute for cookies, cakes, candies, and other foods high in refined sugar. Whole fruit is also beneficial for your body because of its high fiber content. Even though fruit is high in sugar, its high-fiber content helps slow down absorption of the sugar into the blood and thereby helps stabilize the blood sugar level. The fiber content in fruit also helps prevent constipation. I recommend, however, using fruit juices only in small quantities. Fruit juice does not contain the bulk or fiber of the whole fruit and can destabilize your blood sugar level.

Seeds and Nuts. Sesame seeds, sunflower seeds, pistachios, pecans, and almonds are all good sources of non-heme or vegetarian iron. They are also very high in other essential nutrients, such as magnesium, calcium, and fatty acids. Ground flaxseeds (flax meal) contains both lignans and the essential fatty acids, alpha-linolenic and linoleic acid. The lignans help to reduce excessive levels of estrogen in the body, while the flaxseed oil helps reduce irregular and heavy menstrual bleeding by promoting healthy ovulation and the production of progesterone. This was demonstrated in a study at the University of Minnesota.

Combine 4 to 6 tablespoons of ground flax meal with soy or rice milk or a delicious instant cereal. Flaxseeds can be purchased in natural foods stores.

The oils in seeds and nuts are very perishable, so exposure to light, heat, and oxygen should be avoided. Seeds and nuts should be eaten raw and unsalted to get the benefit of their essential fatty acids—which are good for your skin and hair—as well as to avoid the negative effects of too much salt. Whenever possible, purchase unshelled nuts and seeds. If you buy them already shelled, refrigerate them so their oils don't become rancid. Do not buy broken nuts as they become rancid faster and lose their nutrient value. Nuts and seeds make a wonderful garnish on salads, vegetable dishes, and casseroles. They can also be eaten as a main source of protein with snacks and light meals.

Poultry and Fish. Meat is an exceptionally good source of the easily absorbed heme iron. It also contains high levels of other essential nutrients needed to prevent anemia, especially vitamin C, vitamin B12, and folic acid. Meat is also high in other blood builders, including protein, copper, and zinc. Your best meat choices include liver, oysters, trout, scallops, shrimp, poultry, and venison.

If you find meat difficult to digest, you may need to use supplementary digestive enzymes.

If you do include meat in your irregular and heavy menstrual bleeding dietary program, I recommend that you use it in moderate amounts (6 ounces or less per day). Most Americans eat much more protein than is healthy in their diets. Excessive amounts of protein are difficult to digest and stress the kidneys. Except for fish, meat is also a primary source of unhealthy saturated fats which put you at higher risk for heart disease and cancer. Instead of using meat as your only source of protein, I recommend that you increase your intake of grains, beans, and raw seeds and nuts, which contain protein as well as many other important nutrients. I recommend that my patients use meat more as a flavoring for casseroles, stir-fries, and soups. Buy organic, range-fed meat to ensure the animal's exposure to pesticides, antibiotics, and hormones is reduced.

Oils. As discussed on the previous page under *Seeds and Nuts*, flaxseed oil contributes to healthy ovulation and progesterone production in the body which, in turn, helps to limit heavy menstrual bleeding. Use 1 to 2 tablespoons of flaxseed oil each day. Other oils — including wheat germ oil, soybean oil, and corn oil — contain vitamin E, which is an important nutrient for red blood cell survival and helps to regulate menstruation. For menopausal women, oils with high vitamin E content help to suppress hot flashes and moodiness. Wheat germ oil contains the highest levels of vitamin E and, in fact, is the source for most natural vitamin E sold on the market today. Cold-pressed oils tend to be fresher and purer. Keep oils refrigerated to avoid rancidity. Vegetable oils, such as olive oil and sesame oil, can be used in small amounts for cooking, stir-frying, and sautéing. Oils such as flax oil or pumpkin seed oil should not be used for cooking since they are heat sensitive and are altered chemically at high temperatures.

Foods to Avoid with Irregular Menstruation

The following foods should be avoided or at least limited in your diet. These foods can increase the tendency toward both irregular and heavy menstrual bleeding. You will notice that many of these foods are recognized as being stressful and unhealthy for your body in general.

Dairy Products. Women with irregular and heavy menstruation should avoid dairy products. Clinical studies have shown that dairy products decrease iron absorption in anemic women. Their high saturated fat content is a risk factor for promoting excess estrogen levels in the body, a common cause of heavy menstrual bleeding. And this isn't the only bad news. Dairy products have many other unhealthy effects on a woman's body. The tryptophan in milk has a sedative effect that increases fatigue, a real problem for anemic women. Many women are allergic to dairy products or lack the enzymes to digest milk, resulting in digestive problems such as bloating, gas, and bowel changes. Intolerance to dairy products can hamper the absorption and assimilation of the calcium they contain. Dairy products are also high in salt, which can increase bloating and increase the risk of high blood pressure, heart attacks, and strokes.

Women who are concerned about their calcium intake can turn to the many other good dietary sources of this essential nutrient. These include beans, peas, soybeans, sesame seeds, soup stock made from chicken or fish bones, and green leafy vegetables. For food preparation, soy milk, rice milk, and nut milk are excellent substitutions. I also recommend a supplement containing calcium, magnesium, and vitamin D to make sure your intake is sufficient.

Fats. Fat constitutes 40 percent of the calories in the typical American diet. Most of this fat comes from unhealthy saturated sources such as dairy products, red meat, and eggs. This diet tends to promote heavy menstrual bleeding in susceptible women, because excessive saturated fat intake is stressful to the liver and helps to increase excess estrogen levels. This type of fat also puts women at high risk for heart disease and cancer of the breast, uterus, and ovaries. Women on a high-fat diet also tend to accumulate excess weight more easily. Eat more fruits, vegetables, grains, fish, and poultry instead of foods high in saturated fats. As often as possible, eat fresh and homemade foods prepared with a minimum of fats and oils.

If you must eat packaged and processed foods, read the labels and avoid those foods with a high fat content. Red meat should be used only in small amounts. Avoid rich recipes that use large amounts of butter, cream, cheese or other high-fat foods in the preparation. Instead, flavor foods with garlic, onions, herbs, lemon juice, or a little olive oil (a monosaturated fat that doesn't increase your cholesterol level). Eat raw seeds and nuts rather than cooked ones (cooking alters the nature of the oils), and use them sparingly because of their high fat content.

Alcohol. Alcohol should be avoided entirely or consumed only in small amounts by women with heavy menstrual bleeding. Alcohol depletes the body's B-complex vitamins and minerals, which can worsen both heavy and irregular menstruation and anemia. It also disrupts carbohydrate metabolism. Alcohol is toxic to the liver and can affect the liver's ability to metabolize hormones efficiently. Excessive alcohol intake has been associated with lack of ovulation and elevated estrogen levels, which can trigger heavy menstrual bleeding in susceptible women. In large amounts, alcohol can be toxic to the heart and nervous system. When used carefully, not exceeding 4 ounces of wine per day, 10 ounces of beer, or 1 ounce of hard liquor, it can have a delightfully relaxing effect. It makes us more sociable and enhances the taste of food. For optimal health, however, I recommend using alcohol only as an occasional treat, not more than once or twice a week. Women who are particularly susceptible to the negative effects of alcohol shouldn't drink it at all.

If you entertain often and enjoy social drinking, I recommend that you try nonalcoholic beverages. A nonalcoholic cocktail, such as mineral water with a twist of lime or lemon or a dash of bitters, is a good substitute. "Near beer" is a nonalcoholic beer substitute that tastes quite good. Light wine and beer have a lower alcohol content than hard liquor, liqueurs, and regular wine.

Caffeine. Coffee, black tea, soft drinks, and chocolate—all of these foods contain caffeine, a stimulant that many women use to increase their energy level and alertness and to decrease fatigue. Unfortunately, caffeine has many negative effects on the body. Caffeine can worsen hormonal imbalances in women. When used in excess, it also increases anxiety, irritability, and mood swings. This can be a real problem for women with irregular and heavy menstruation and anemia who have lowered emotional and physical reserves. Caffeine also depletes the body's stores of B-complex vitamins. This interferes with carbohydrate metabolism and healthy liver function, which helps to regulate estrogen levels and menstrual bleeding.

Many menopausal women also complain that caffeine increases the frequency of hot flashes. Coffee, black tea, chocolate, and soft drinks all act to inhibit iron absorption. Black tea contains tannins that inhibit iron absorption; particularly when a meal is deficient in vitamin C. Polyphenols found in coffee also interfere with iron absorption, as do the oxalic acid found in chocolate and the additives in soft drinks. Caffeinated foods and beverages should be avoided by a woman with irregular and heavy menstruation and anemia.

Considering all of these negative effects, women should either cut down dramatically on caffeine intake or eliminate it entirely. Because cutting out caffeine can cause withdrawal symptoms such as irritability and headaches, I recommend that women eliminate caffeine gradually. To start, mix half a cup of regular coffee with half a cup of decaffeinated coffee. I recommend using water-processed decaffeinated coffee, which is extracted with hot water rather than chemicals. After a month or two on decaffeinated coffee, switch to grain-based coffee substitutes, such as Postum or Cafix. Because they have a calming effect, herbal teas made from chamomile and hops can actually be therapeutic for women with anxiety.

Sugar. Like alcohol, sugar depletes the body's B-complex vitamins and minerals, which can increase nervous tension and anxiety (real problems for anemic women). Unfortunately, most Americans eat too much sugar — the average American eats 120 pounds per year. Sugar addiction is very common in our society in people of all ages. Many people use sweet foods as a way to deal with their frustrations and other upsets. Many convenience foods, including salad dressing, catsup, and relish, contain high levels of both sugar and salt. Sugar is the main ingredient in soft drinks and in desserts such as candies, cookies, cakes, and ice cream. Foods high in sugar content also lead to tooth loss through tooth decay and gum disease. Of even greater significance is the fact that excessive sugar intake can have a negative effect on diabetes and blood sugar imbalances.

Try to satisfy your sweet tooth instead with healthier foods, such as fruit or grain-based desserts like oatmeal cookies sweetened with fruit or honey. You will find that small amounts of these foods can satisfy your cravings. Instead of disrupting your mood and energy level, they actually have a healthful and balancing effect.

Salt. While not directly contributing to heavy menstrual bleeding, excessive salt intake should be avoided. Too much dietary salt can increase high blood pressure, bloating, and fluid retention, and can contribute to osteoporosis in menopausal women. Unfortunately, large amounts of salt are commonly found in the American diet as table salt (sodium chloride),

MSG (monosodium glutamate), and a variety of food additives. Fast foods such as hamburgers, hot dogs, french fries, pizza, and tacos are loaded with salt and saturated fats. Common processed foods such as soups, potato chips, cheese, olives, salad dressings, and catsup (to name only a few) are also very high in salt. To make matters worse, many people add too much salt while cooking and seasoning their meals.

For women of all ages, I recommend eliminating added salt in your meals. For flavor, use seasonings like garlic, herbs, spices, and lemon juice. Avoid processed foods that are high in salt, including canned foods, olives, pickles, potato chips, tortilla chips, catsup, and salad dressings. Many frozen entrees are also too high in salt and fat content. Learn to read labels and look for the word sodium (table salt). If it appears high on the list of ingredients, don't buy the product. Many items in health food stores are labeled "no salt added." Some supermarkets offer "no added salt" foods in their diet or health food sections.

Substitute Healthy Ingredients in Recipes

Over the years of working in nutritional medicine, I have found it easy to adapt many "forbidden recipes" to the needs of my own nutritional program. These high-stress recipes would start out filled with ingredients I couldn't normally eat—fats, dairy products, chocolate, and sugar. By eliminating the high-stress ingredients and replacing them with healthier, more nutritious substitutes, I could still make almost any recipe in my files. I have recommended this technique for years to my patients, who are delighted to find that they can still have their favorite dishes, but in much healthier versions. This is particularly important for women with heavy menstrual bleeding, since proper dietary intake can play a major role in the healing process.

One method of modifying your diet is to totally eliminate the chocolate, milk products, sugar, salt, and other high-stress ingredients that many recipes call for. These items are not necessary to make foods taste good, and they can worsen your symptoms. If you want to retain a high-stress ingredient, you can substantially reduce the amount you use, and still retain the flavor and taste. Most of us have palates jaded by too much salt, fat, sugar, and other flavorings. In many dishes, we taste only the additives; we never really enjoy the delicious flavor of the foods themselves. Now that I make a habit of substituting low-stress ingredients in my cooking, I find that I enjoy the subtle taste of the dishes much more. Also, I find that my health and vitality continue to improve with the deletion of high-stress ingredients from my food. The following information tells you how to substitute healthy ingredients in your own recipes. The substitutions are simple to make and should benefit your health greatly.

How to Substitute for Dairy Products

Use soy cheese in food preparation and cooking. Soy cheese is an excellent substitute for cow's milk cheese. It is lower in fat and salt, and the fat that it contains isn't saturated. There are many brands available in health food stores, as well as many different flavors — mozzarella, cheddar, American, and jack. The quality of these products keeps improving all the time. You can use soy cheese as a perfect cheese substitute in sandwiches, salads, pizzas, lasagnas, and casseroles.

Decrease the amount of cow's milk cheese you use in food preparation and cooking. If you must use cow's milk cheese in cooking, decrease the amount by one-half to two-thirds so that it becomes a flavoring or garnish, rather than a major source of fat and protein. Soft tofu can be added to the recipes to replace the volume of cheese you have omitted. I have done this often with lasagna, layering the lasagna noodles with tofu and topping with melted soy cheese for a delicious dish. The tofu, which is bland, takes on the taste of the tomato sauce. If you cannot give up cow's milk products, try to use the lower-fat cheese now available. Goat's or sheep's milk cheese in small amounts can also be used to replace taste of the tomato sauce. If you cannot give up cow's milk products, try to use the lower-fat cheese now available. Goat's or sheep's milk cheese in small amounts can also be used to replace cow's milk cheese, since the fat they contain is more easily emulsified in the body.

Milk can often be easily replaced in recipes. Substitute potato milk, soy milk, nut milk, or grain milk for cow's milk. Soy milk and nut milk are available at most health food stores. Soy milk is particularly good and comes in many flavors. Many nondairy types of milk are good sources of calcium and can be used for drinking, eating, or baking. (See Chapter 7 for an easy way to make an almond-based milk substitute.) Three glasses of soy milk each day contains enough of the weak estrogen-like substances called isoflavones to help reduce excess estrogen levels within the body. Use with other sources of soy like tofu or soy-based burgers and hot dogs.

Substitute flax oil for butter. Flax oil is the best substitute for butter that I have found. It is a golden, rich oil that looks and tastes quite a bit like butter. It is delicious on anything you would normally top with butter—toast, rice, popcorn, steamed vegetables, and potatoes. Flax oil is extremely high in essential fatty acids—the type of fat that is very healthy for a woman's body. Essential fatty acids help promote normal hormonal function. Flax oil is quite perishable, however, because it is sensitive to heat and light. You cannot cook with it—cook the food first and add the flax oil before serving. It also needs to be refrigerated. There are so many health benefits to flax oil that I recommend it highly. You can find it in health food stores.

How to Substitute for Caffeinated Foods and Beverages

Drink substitutes for coffee and black tea. For cooking, try the grain-based coffee substitutes, such as Postum and Cafix.

Use decaffeinated coffee or tea as a transition beverage. For women who cannot give up coffee, start by substituting water-processed decaffeinated coffee for the real thing. Then try to wean yourself from coffee altogether, or drink a coffee substitute.

Use herbal teas for energy and vitality. Many women drink coffee simply for the pickup they get from it. Their cups of coffee in the morning enable them to wake up and function through the day. Use ginger instead. It is a great herbal stimulant that won't wreck your health. See recipe section for instructions on how to make ginger tea.

Substitute carob for chocolate. Unsweetened carob tastes like chocolate but is far more nutritious. A member of the legume family, carob is high in calcium. It can be purchased in chunk form as a substitute for chocolate candy, or as a powder to be used in baking or drinks. Be careful, however, not to overindulge; carob, like chocolate, is high in calories and fat. It should be considered a treat and a cooking aid to be used only in small amounts.

How to Substitute for Sugar

Cut the amount of sweetener in your recipes by one-third to one-half Americans tend to be addicted to sugar. Most of us grew up on highly sugared soft drinks, candy, and rich pastries—no wonder the incidence of diabetes is soaring among our population. I have found that as women decrease their sugar intake, most of them begin to really enjoy the subtle flavors of the foods they eat.

Substitute more concentrated sweeteners. Concentrated sweeteners such as honey and maple syrup have a sweeter taste per quantity used than table sugar. Using these substitutes will allow you to decrease the actual amount of sweetener in a recipe. If you use a concentrated sweetener in place of sugar in an ordinary recipe, reduce the liquid content in the recipe by one-fourth cup. If no liquid is used in the recipe, add 3 to 5 tablespoons of flour for each three-fourths cup of concentrated sweetener.

Substitute fruit for sugar in pastries. In making muffins and cookies, you may want to try deleting sugar altogether and adding extra fruits and nuts.

How to Substitute for Salt

Substitute potassium-based products for table salt (sodium chloride). Potassium-based products are much healthier and will not aggravate heart disease or hypertension.

Use powdered seaweeds such as kelp or nori to season vegetables, grains, and salads. They are high in essential iodine and trace elements.

Use herbs instead of salt for flavoring. Their flavors are much more subtle and will help even the most jaded palate appreciate the taste of fresh fruits, vegetables, and meats.

Use liquid flavoring agents with advertised low-sodium content. Low-salt soy sauce and Bragg's Amino Acids, a liquid soybean-based flavoring agent, are delicious when used as salt substitutes in cooking. Add them to soups, casseroles, stir-fries, and other dishes at the end of the cooking process. You will find that you need only a small amount for intense flavoring.

How to Substitute for White Flour (Wheat Based)

Use whole grain, non-wheat flour. White flour loses most of its nutrient content through processing. Substitute whole grain flour, which is much higher in essential nutrients, including the B-complex vitamins and many minerals. It is also higher in fiber content.

Use rice flour or barley flour as a wheat substitute. Rice flour makes excellent cookies, cakes, and other pastries. Barley flour is best used for pie crusts.

How to Substitute for Alcohol

Use low-alcohol or nonalcoholic products for cooking. Substitute low-alcohol or nonalcoholic wine or beer when cooking or preparing sauces and marinades. Much of the flavor that alcohol imparts will be retained, and the stress factor will decrease substantially.

Substitutes for Common High-Stress Ingredients

3/4 cup sugar	3/4 cup xylitol
	1/2 cup honey
	1/4 cup molasses
	1/2 cup maple syrup
	1/2 ounce barley malt
	1 cup apple butter
	2 cups apple juice
1 cup milk	1 cup soy, rice, nut, or grain milk
1 tablespoon butter	1 tablespoon flax oil (must be used raw and unheated)
1/2 teaspoon salt	1 tablespoon miso
	1/2 teaspoon potassium chloride salt substitute
	1/2 teaspoon Mrs. Dash, Spike
	1/2 teaspoon herbs (basil, tarragon, oregano, etc.)
1 1/2 cups cocoa	1 cup powdered carob
1 square chocolate	3/4 tablespoon powdered carob
1 tablespoon coffee	1 tablespoon decaffeinated coffee
	1 tablespoon Postum, Cafix, or other grain-based coffee substitute
4 ounces wine	4 ounces light wine
8 ounces beer	8 ounces near beer
1 cup white flour	1 cup barley flour (pie crust)
	1 cup rice flour (cookies, cakes, breads)

Healthy Food Shopping List

Vegetables

Beets
Bok choy
Broccoli
Brussels sprouts
Cabbage
Carrots
Cauliflower
Celery
Chard
Cilantro
Collard
Cucumbers
Dandelion greens

Eggplant
Garlic
Green beans
Horseradish
Kale
Lettuce
Mustard greens
Okra
Onions
Parsley
Parsnips
Peas (all varieties)
Potatoes

Radicchio
Radishes
Rutabagas
Sauerkraut
Spinach
Squash
Sweet potatoes
Tomatoes
Turnips
Turnip greens
Watercress
Yams

Legumes
Adzuki
Black
Black-eyed peas
Cannellini
Fava
Garbanzo
Kidney
Lentils
Navy
Red
Soy: tofu, tempeh
Turtle beans

Whole Grains
Amaranth
Barley
Brown rice
Buckwheat
Corn
Millet
Oatmeal
Quinoa
Rye

Seeds and Nuts
Almonds
Cashews
Filberts
Flaxseeds
Macadamia
Pecan
Pumpkin seeds
Sesame seeds
Sunflower seeds
Walnuts

Healthy Food Shopping List (continued)

Fruits
Acai berries
Apples
Avocado
Bananas
Berries
Blueberries
Raspberries
Strawberries
Coconuts
Goji berries
Kiwi
Noni
Olives
Pomegranates
Pears
Seasonal fruits

Sweeteners
Brown rice syrup
Honey
Maple syrup
Molasses
Stevia
Xylitol

Beverages
Coconut water
Grain based coffee
substitute
Herbal tea
Green tea
Water

Meats
Fish
Free-range poultry
Game meat
Organic lean red meat
Seafood (in
moderation)

Oils
Flax
Macadamia
Olive
Safflower
Sesame
Walnut

**Foods from other
cultures**
Gomasio
Jicama
Miso
Seaweed (like kelp,
dulse, nori, wakane)
Tamari soy sauce
Umeboshi plums

Dairy Substitutes
Hemp milk
Nut milk
Rice milk
Soy milk
Soy, coconut, almond,
rice or hemp cheeses,
cream cheese, yogurt,
and frozen desserts
*Avoid all soy products
containing
hydrogenated oil.

Herbs & Spices
Basil
Black pepper
Cayenne pepper
Chamomile
Chili pepper, dried
Cilantro
Cinnamon, ground
Cloves
Coriander
Cumin
Dill
Ginger
Licorice
Mustard seeds
Oregano
Peppermint
Poppy
Rosemary
Sage
Tarragon
Thyme
Turmeric

6

Menus, Meal Plans & Recipes

Many of my patients with irregular and heavy menstrual bleeding have asked me for specific recipes and meal plans to help optimize their healing program. Unfortunately, there are very few of these specific resources available for women. For instance, no cookbooks adequately address a woman's needs for specific nutrients. Most cookbooks have dishes that look and taste great but are laden with ingredients that can actually worsen a woman's condition—including such high-stress foods as dairy products, fats, chocolate, sugar, and caffeinated beverages. Some recent cookbooks do present low-calorie "light dishes." Although these cookbooks eliminate fats and sugars from the recipes, they still don't give women with heavy menstrual bleeding the therapeutic levels of specific nutrients they require.

To answer this need, I have developed a number of meal plans and recipes specifically for women with irregular and heavy menstrual bleeding. Not only have the recipes been designed to look and taste good, but they contain high levels of the nutrients you need to help rebuild and repair your body as well as those needed to help prevent heavy menstrual bleeding.

The recipes I have included in this chapter are quick and easy to prepare. Most women have very busy lives, and I have found that anything too complicated won't work for me or my patients. Best of all, these recipes are delicious and satisfying as well as healthful. I hope that you enjoy them as much as I do.

Menus

Breakfast Menus

These breakfast menus have been developed to help reduce and prevent symptoms of endometriosis. All the dishes contain high levels of the essential nutrients that women with these problems need; the recipes call for no high-stress ingredients. You can use these as idea generators for your own meal planning.

Breakfast has been one of the easiest meals for my patients to restructure along healthier lines. It tends to be a smaller and simpler meal. You may want to make healthful dietary changes in your breakfast first and then move on to lunch and dinner.

Flax shake with protein powder
and fresh fruit
~~~~~~~~~~~~~~
Blueberry and green food smoothie
~~~~~~~~~~~~~~
Millet cereal with raisins and
cinnamon
Nondairy yogurt
Chamomile tea
~~~~~~~~~~~~~~
Rice and flaxseed pancakes
Banana
Vanilla nondairy milk
~~~~~~~~~~~~~~

Oatmeal with raspberries
Chamomile tea
~~~~~~~~~~~~~~
Nondairy yogurt with granola
and ground flaxseed
Peppermint tea
~~~~~~~~~~~~~~
Gluten-free waffles with maple
syrup and sliced bananas
Ginger tea
~~~~~~~~~~~~~~
Corn muffins
Raw sesame seed butter
Roasted grain beverage (coffee
substitute)
~~~~~~~~~~~~~~

Lunch and Dinner Menus

Here is a variety of menus you can choose from when planning your meals. You can use these menu plans or as idea generators to fit your own taste and needs. These dishes contain many nutritious and healthful ingredients for endometriosis relief. Use these menus as helpful guidelines throughout the entire month. Your nutritional status on a day-by-day basis determines in part how likely you are to have endometriosis symptoms. These dishes should help to diminish the severity of your symptoms because they eliminate high-stress foods.

Soup Meals

Split pea soup
Corn muffins
Fresh applesauce
~~~~~~~~~~~~~~
Chicken and wild rice soup
Cole slaw
Millet bread with flax oil
~~~~~~~~~~~~~~
Vegetable soup with brown rice
Steamed kale
Baked potato with flax oil
Apple slices
~~~~~~~~~~~~~~
Lentil soup
Herbed brown rice
Broccoli with lemon
~~~~~~~~~~~~~~
Tomato soup
Potato salad with low-fat mayonnaise
Celery and carrot sticks
~~~~~~~~~~~~~~

Salad Meals

Spinach salad with turkey bacon or tofu
Corn muffins with flax oil
Orange slices
~~~~~~~~~~~~~~
Beet salad with goat cheese
Rice crackers with fresh fruit preserves
~~~~~~~~~~~~~~
Romaine salad with grilled salmon
Gluten-free bread and olive oil dip
~~~~~~~~~~~~~~
Low-fat potato salad
Cole slaw
Hard boiled eggs
Melon slices
~~~~~~~~~~~~~~
Mixed Vegetable Salad with Kidney Beans
Baked yam

Meat Meals

Poached salmon with lemon
Herbed brown rice
Steamed carrots with honey
~~~~~~~~~~~~~~

Roasted chicken with herbs
Baked potato with flax oil
Broccoli with lemon
~~~~~~~~~~~~~~

Broiled trout with dill
Mixed green salad with vinaigrette
Green peas and onions
Apple slices
~~~~~~~~~~~~~~

Grilled shrimp with olive oil and
lemon
Wild rice
Steamed kale
~~~~~~~~~~~~~~

One-Dish Vegetable Meals

Vegetarian tacos with black beans,
brown rice, avocados, tomatoes,
lettuce and low-salt salsa
~~~~~~~~~~~~~~

Stir-fry with mixed vegetables,
brown rice and tofu
Orange slices
~~~~~~~~~~~~~~

Pasta with tomato sauce, broccoli,
carrots, olive oil and garlic
Green salad with vinaigrette
~~~~~~~~~~~~~~

Hummus dip
Eggplant dip (babaganoush)
Mixed raw vegetable slices
including carrots, red bell peppers,
and radishes
~~~~~~~~~~~~~~

Brown rice and almond tabouli
Mixed olives
Melon slices
~~~~~~~~~~~~~~

Breakfast Recipes

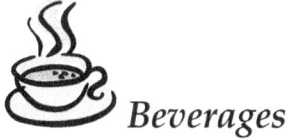 *Beverages*

These drinks are made with therapeutic herbal teas,, power smoothies that are rich in fruits, raw seeds, nuts, protein powder, green foods and non dairy milk that are recommended for preventing and treating your symptoms. The ingredients contain high levels of essential nutrients that help regulate your hormonal balance and relax tension in the muscles of the pelvis and lower extremities. You can enjoy these beverages throughout the month, and not just during your symptom time, as their high mineral and other nutrient content is beneficial for the entire body.

Relaxant Herb Tea   Serves 2

2 cups water
1 teaspoon chamomile leaves
1 teaspoon peppermint leaves
1 teaspoon honey (if desired)

Bring the water to a boil. Place herbs in water and stir. Turn heat to low and simmer for 15 minutes.

Peppermint and chamomile are both muscle relaxants and antispasmodic herbs, so they can provide relief of pain and cramping caused by endometriosis. They also help calm the mood.

Ginger Tea   Serves 4

Ginger makes a warming, delicious tea and is beneficial to your circulation. It is also a powerful anti-inflammatory herb. If the tea is too strong add more water.

5 cups water
3 tablespoons ginger coarsely chopped
½ lemon (optional)

Honey (or other sweetener, to taste)

Add ginger to the water in a cooking pot. Bring to a boil and then turn heat to low. Steep for 15 or 20 minutes. Squeeze lemon into tea and serve with honey or your favorite sweetener.

Blueberry Pomegranate Smoothie **Serves 2**

¼ cup nondairy yogurt, unsweetened
¾ cup pomegranate juice
1 cup blueberries, fresh or frozen
1 tablespoon ground flaxseed
1 banana

Combine all ingredients in a blender. Puree until smooth and serve.

.

Raspberry Flax Smoothie   **Serves 2**

This creamy smoothie makes a great breakfast. Flaxseed oil one is my favorite foods. It is both delicious and rich in healthy omega-3 fatty acids. It also adds extra creaminess to the smoothie.

1 cup rice milk
⅔ cup raspberries – fresh or frozen
1 heaping tablespoon rice protein powder
1 tablespoon flaxseed oil
2 bananas, sliced

Combine all ingredients in a blender. Puree until smooth and serve.

Delicious Green Drink   **Serves 1**

½ cup Concord grape juice
¼ cup water
1 tablespoon ground flaxseed
½ teaspoon chlorella powder
½ teaspoon spirulina powder

Mix all ingredients together in a glass or puree in a blender.

Heavenly Strawberry Coconut Smoothie   **Serves 2**

This drink fits its name! It is absolutely scrumptious as well as good for you. If you don't have a high-speed blender and you are using whole raw cashews I recommend that you chop them up beforehand. Otherwise, raw cashew butter is a good substitute.

1 cup coconut milk, unsweetened
1 cup strawberries – fresh or frozen
1 tablespoon raw coconut flour
1 tablespoon raw cashews (about cashews 10-15)
1 banana, sliced

Combine all ingredients in a blender. Puree until smooth and serve.

Simple Flax Smoothie   **Serves 2**

Flaxseed is not only a tasty addition to smoothies but it is also very nutritious. Flaxseed is high in essential fatty acids, calcium, magnesium, and potassium.

1 cup vanilla nondairy milk
2 tablespoons ground flaxseed
1 banana

Combine all ingredients in a blender. Blend until smooth and serve.

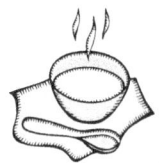 *Healthy, Quick Breakfasts*

Most American breakfasts include wheat and dairy products, such as yogurt, wheat toast, wheat cereal with milk, sweet rolls, and other wheat-based pastries. As I explained in Chapter 4, dairy products and wheat can worsen the symptoms of endometriosis and PMS (which often occurs concurrently).

I have included in this section both whole grain, carbohydrate based entrees as well as protein-rich dishes. depending on the type of diet that makes you feel your best. Both types of entrees, however, will benefit endometriosis symptoms by eliminating wheat and dairy products at breakfast.

The whole grain dishes are based on ground flaxseed, soy, and gluten-free grains, all of which can be useful in reducing your symptoms. The protein-rich entrees have been created using eggs and healthy breakfast meats, Gluten is the protein found in wheat that can trigger symptoms of bloating, digestive disturbances, and fatigue.

Quinoa Cereal with Blueberries   **Serves 2**

1 ½ cups cooked quinoa
1 cup nondairy milk
½ cup blueberries
2 teaspoons honey or other sweetener

Combine quinoa and nondairy milk in a saucepan. Simmer for 5 minutes. Stir in honey and garnish with raspberries.

Quinoa with Prunes **Serves 2**

This is one of my all-time favorite hot cereals. The plums are delicious and add a nice texture. Quinoa is a small, protein rich grain. When cooked the grains are small and fluffy. I recommend making a pot of quinoa the night before.

1 ½ cups cooked quinoa
1 cup nondairy milk
4-6 dried prunes, chopped
2 tablespoons flaxseed oil
2 teaspoons xylitol, honey, or maple syrup (if using unsweetened milk)
Pinch of salt (optional)

In a saucepan combine quinoa, nondairy milk, salt, and dried plums. Heat thoroughly and simmer on low heat for 5-10 minutes until plums have softened. Serve with flaxseed oil and sweetener.

Maple Cinnamon Oatmeal **Serves 2**

1 cup quick oats
1 ¾ cups water
1-2 tablespoons flaxseed oil
2 teaspoons maple syrup
Pinch of cinnamon (to taste)
Pinch of salt

Boil water in a saucepan. Add oats and reduce to medium heat. Cook for one minute and stir. Cover, and remove oatmeal from heat. Serve in 2-3 minutes.

Stir in maple syrup, flaxseed oil, cinnamon and salt.

Strawberries and Cream Oatmeal **Serves 2**

1 cup quick oats
½ cup strawberries, chopped
½ nondairy milk
1 ¼ cups water

1-2 tablespoons flaxseed oil
2 teaspoons honey or stevia
Pinch of salt (optional)

Bring water and nondairy milk to a boil in a saucepan. Add oats and reduce to medium heat. Cook for one minute and stir. Cover, and remove oatmeal from heat. Serve in 2-3 minutes. Stir in sweetener, flaxseed oil, salt and top with strawberries.

Apple Almond Muffins   **Makes 14-18**

The cinnamon and apples in these muffins makes the kitchen smell delicious and welcoming. If you are eating a nut-free diet simply omit the nuts.

2 cups rice flour
1 apple, diced (Granny Smith apple preferred)
½ cup applesauce
6 packets of Truvia (equal to ¼ cup sugar)
1 tablespoon honey
½ cup water
1 egg
3 tablespoons safflower oil
⅓ cup chopped almonds
1 teaspoon cinnamon
¼ teaspoon nutmeg
1 teaspoon baking powder
½ teaspoon baking soda
1/8 teaspoon salt

Preheat oven to 400 degrees. Mix all dry ingredients and wet ingredients separately. Combine and pour a large spoonful (approximately a heaping tablespoon) into each muffin cup. I recommend using baking cups for this recipe.

Bake for 20 minutes until cooked through.

Pumpkin Muffins   **Makes 14-18 muffins**

1½ cups rice flour
½ teaspoon baking powder
½ teaspoon baking soda
1 cup pumpkin
1 teaspoon cinnamon
¼ teaspoon nutmeg
¼ cup chopped almonds (optional)
3 tablespoons molasses
3 tablespoons safflower oil
½ cup raisins
2 eggs
½ cup nondairy milk
1 teaspoon vanilla extract
1/8 teaspoon salt

Preheat oven to 400 degrees. Line a muffin tin with paper muffin cups.

Combine all dry ingredients and mix thoroughly. In a separate bowl beat the two eggs and then combine the remainder of the wet ingredients. Add the wet ingredients to the dry and mix thoroughly.

Fill muffin cups ⅔ with the batter. Cook for 18-20 minutes or until thoroughly cooked.

Flaxseed Pancakes   **Makes 8 pancakes (serves 2-4)**

Xylitol is an excellent sugar substitute for cooking and baking that can be found at most health food stores. Xylitol is easy to use because it has a 1:1 ratio with sugar. Yet, this product has 40% fewer calories than sugar and is beneficial for your teeth and gums.

1 cup gluten-free flour
1 cup unsweetened rice milk
1 egg
2 tablespoons xylitol
1 tablespoon ground flaxseed

1 teaspoon baking powder
½ teaspoon baking soda
¼ teaspoon salt
3 tablespoons almond oil, keeping 1 tbsp. for cooking
Maple syrup (optional)
Fruit jam (optional)

Mix the dry and wet ingredients in separate bowls. Combine all the ingredients and mix thoroughly. Cook on medium heat and use a small amount of oil to grease the pan if needed. When pancakes bubble in the center flip and cook for 1-2 minutes until cooked thoroughly. Serve with maple syrup or all-fruit jam. Delicious!

Egg and Sausage Scramble   **Serves 2**

4 eggs
4 turkey breakfast sausages
2 slice of gluten free toast
Salt and pepper (optional)
2 teaspoons olive oil
Serve with ½ cup applesauce

Warm a frying pan on medium heat and add olive oil. Beat egg gently in a small bowl and set aside. Chop the sausages into small pieces - this will help them to cook faster. Add sausages to the pan and cook for several minutes until sausages are brown. Turn heat to low and add eggs to the pan and scramble with the sausage. Add a pinch of salt and pepper. Serve with toast and applesauce.

Bake for 20-25 minutes until cooked through.

Red Pepper and Sausage Wrap   **Serves 2**

2 brown rice tortillas
½ cup red pepper, diced
⅓ cup onion, diced
3 eggs, beaten
2 turkey breakfast sausages, cut into small pieces
1 tablespoon olive oil
Salt and pepper – generous pinch

In a frying pan on medium heat the olive oil. Add the sausage and cook until lightly browned. Add the onions and red peppers and cook until onions begin to soften, about 2 minutes. Next, add eggs and salt and pepper. Let eggs sit until they begin to cook slightly and then scramble.

Lightly warm the tortillas and put the egg scramble into the tortillas. Top the eggs with one tablespoon of salsa.

Spinach and Tomato Scramble   **Serves 2**

The Parmesan cheese adds a delightful saltiness and tang to this dish.

4 eggs, beaten
1 tablespoon water
2 tablespoons diced onion
¼ tomato, chopped
12 spinach leaves, chopped
1 tablespoon olive oil
Salt and Pepper (optional)
Parmesan cheese - or soy Parmesan (optional)

Beat the 4 eggs together with 1 tablespoon water. Preheat the frying pan on medium heat and add 1 tablespoon olive oil. Add onion and cook for about 3 minutes until onions are translucent. Next add eggs, spinach and tomato. Let sit for about 15 seconds and then start to scramble with your spatula. Sprinkle on a small amount of Parmesan cheese, add a pinch of salt and pepper and serve

83   The Irregular Menstruation Cure

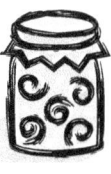 *Spreads and Sauces*

These spreads and sauces contain highly concentrated levels of ingredients that help to relax endometriosis-related pain and muscle tension and help to relieve congestion. Serve with rice cakes, crackers, corn bread, or even spread on a banana for a delicious treat.

Fresh Applesauce   **Serves 2**

2 ½ apples
½ cup fresh apple juice
½ teaspoon cinnamon
½ teaspoon ginger

Peel apples and cut into quarters; remove cores. Combine all ingredients in a food processor. Blend until smooth.

Sesame-Tofu Spread   **Serves 4**

¼ cup soft tofu
¼ cup raw sesame butter
¼ cup honey

Combine all ingredients in a blender. Serve with rice cakes or crackers.

Lunch and Dinner Recipes

These high-nutrient, healthful lunch and dinner dishes are designed to help prevent and relieve your symptoms. The ingredients do not include red meat, dairy products, or wheat, all of which can worsen your symptoms. Mix and match these dishes as you please. You might combine soups and salads or whole grains, legumes and vegetables for a complete vegetarian emphasis or meat based meal., depending on your needs for carbohydrates and protein.

The main course dishes are all extremely healthful for women with endometriosis. You can enjoy these dishes particularly during the second half of your menstrual cycle when your symptoms are worse, but for optimal health and well-being, I recommend their use all month long.

 *Soups*

Chicken Rice Soup   **Serves 4-6**

Few things make me feel better than a bowl of homemade chicken rice soup. I have an easy tip to add extra flavor to your soup: If you used the meat from a roasted, skin-on chicken you can add some of the skin to the soup while it is cooking. This will add depth and richness to your soup. Remove the skin when the soup has finished cooking.

6 cups low-sodium chicken broth
⅔ cup carrot
1 cup celery, diced
1 cup cooked chicken, diced
⅔ cup onion, diced
⅔ cup brown rice, cooked
Tamari soy sauce – to taste (optional)

Bring water to a boil and add all ingredients. Reduce heat to low and simmer for 30 minutes, stirring occasionally. If water begins to cook off add up to an extra cup of water. Add a dash of tamari soy sauce for a saltier flavor.

Split Pea Soup   **Serves 4**

¾ cup split peas
5 cups low-sodium chicken broth
⅔ cup carrot, chopped
¾ cup onion, diced
Tamari soy sauce – to taste (optional)

Bring the water to a boil and add the split peas, onion, carrots, and chicken broth. Reduce heat to low and simmer for 50 minutes – 1 hour, stirring occasionally. If water begins to cook off add up to an extra cup of water. Add a dash of tamari soy sauce for a saltier flavor. .

Black Bean Soup   **Serves 4**

This recipe is easy and makes a delicious, filling soup.

1 can black beans (14 ounce), rinsed
5 cups low-sodium vegetable broth
1 cup onion, diced
⅔ cup carrot, chopped
⅔ cup red pepper, chopped
¼ teaspoon cumin
Tamari soy sauce – to taste (optional)

Bring the water to a boil and add all ingredients. Reduce heat to low and simmer for 30 minutes, stirring occasionally. If water begins to cook off add up to an extra cup of water. Add a dash of tamari soy sauce for a saltier flavor.

Butternut Squash Soup Serves 4

This soup has been a long-time favorite of mine. I adore the light, creamy texture. Adding maple syrup enhances the natural sweetness of the squash.

½ onion, diced
1 cup low-sodium chicken broth
2 cups pureed butternut squash - fresh or frozen (fresh is preferred)
½ teaspoon cinnamon
1½ cups nondairy milk
2 tablespoons maple syrup
1 tablespoon safflower oil
½-¾ teaspoon salt

In a large saucepan heat the oil on medium heat. Add the onion and cook until translucent. Add the butternut squash, chicken broth, cinnamon and salt. Mix well and simmer for 5 minutes. Add nondairy milk and maple syrup. Simmer on low heat for ten minutes. Stir frequently while cooking the soup. *Optional*: To make extra creamy, blend the soup when it has finished cooking. Wait for the soup to cool before blending.

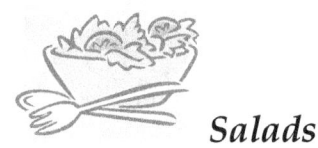 *Salads*

Zingy Watercress Salad   **Serves 4**

I enjoy the refreshing bitterness of watercress. This salad pairs well with green apple. Watercress has a strong flavor and a little goes a long way.

1 cup watercress, coarsely chopped
4 cups butter lettuce (or other soft lettuce), coarsely chopped
2 teaspoons scallions, finely chopped
½ green apple, chopped
1 ounce goat cheese, crumbled
Vinaigrette dressing (see recipe)

In a large bowl toss the watercress, butter lettuce, green onion, and apple together with the vinaigrette dressing (to taste). On top of the salad crumble the goat cheese.

.

Caesar Salad   **Serves 2-4**

I love Caesar salads. They have been my favorite salad for years! The crispy romaine lettuce and creamy dressing is a perfect match. I like to use anchovies because they are delicious in this salad and also full of healthy anti-inflammatory oils. I prefer the filets packed in olive oil.

1 head of romaine lettuce, chopped – about 6 cups
4 tablespoons light Caesar dressing
4 anchovy filets, chopped
⅔ cup gluten free croutons (see recipe)
1½ teaspoons grated Parmesan cheese
1 cup roast chicken, cubed (optional)

In a large mixing bowl pour Caesar's dressing over lettuce. Mix well so that leaves are evenly coated with dressing. Add croutons, Parmesan cheese, anchovies, and toss well. Top with roasted chicken and serve.

Classic Spinach Salad   Serves 4

My tip for cooking great turkey bacon is to cook it on medium-low heat. It takes a few extra minutes but is definitely worth it!

1 bunch of spinach, approximately 6 cups
4 slices of turkey bacon, cooked crisp and crumbled
2 eggs, sliced or chopped
½ cup red pepper, chopped
¼ red onion, sliced very thin
¾ cup mushrooms, sliced thin
Balsamic-Honey Dressing or Raspberry Honey Dressing (see recipes)

In a large bowl place the bacon, egg, red pepper, onion, and mushrooms on top of the spinach. Before serving toss the salad and

Scrumptious Veggie Salad   Serves 4-6

This is one of my favorite salads! It pairs wonderfully with soups and sandwiches

1 head red lettuce, chopped into bite size pieces
1 large tomato, chopped
2 green onions, sliced
6 mushrooms, sliced
¾ cup kidney beans – canned works well
1 avocado, sliced
¼ cup sunflower seeds
Vinaigrette dressing (to taste)

Combine all ingredients except for avocado in a large salad bowl. Mix in Vinaigrette Dressing and top with avocado slices before serving.

Radicchio and Orange Salad   **Serves 4-6**

This is a sophisticated and delicious salad. I love salads with "extras" such as fruit or a little bit of goat cheese.

6 cups salad greens
½ radicchio, sliced thin
⅓ red onion, sliced very thin
3 ounces goat cheese
1 medium sized orange, peeled and cut into bite size segments
Orange vinaigrette (see recipe)

In a large bowl combine salad greens, radicchio, onion, and oranges. Pour vinaigrette, to taste, over salad and toss. Add goat cheese before serving.

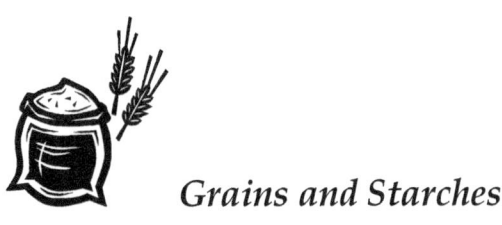 *Grains and Starches*

Wild Rice   Serves 2

⅔ cup wild rice
2 ½ cups water
½ teaspoon sea salt

Wash rice with cold water. Combine all ingredients in a cooking pot and bring to a rapid boil. Turn flame to low, cover, and cook without stirring (about 45 minutes) until rice is tender but not mushy. Uncover and fluff with a fork. Cook an additional 5 minutes, and then serve.

Kasha   Serves 4

1 cup kasha (buckwheat groats)
3 ¼ cups water
Pinch salt

Bring ingredients to a boil, lower heat, and simmer for 25 minutes or until soft. The grains should be fluffy, like rice. *For breakfast, blend in blender with water until creamy. Add almond milk, sesame milk, or sunflower milk, and cinnamon, apple butter, raisins, or berries.*

Delicious Baked Sweet Potato   Serves 4

4 sweet potatoes
1 teaspoon olive oil
1 tablespoon flax oil for each potato

Preheat oven to 400° F. Wash the potatoes, then rub with olive oil. Bake for 45 to 60 minutes, or until soft when pierced with a fork. Garnish with flax oil. Honey, maple syrup, or chopped raw pecans may also be used.

Baked Potato   **Serves 4**

4 russet or Idaho potatoes
2 teaspoons olive oil
1 tablespoon flax oil for each potato

Preheat oven to 400° F. Wash the potatoes, rub them with olive oil, and bake for 45 to 60 minutes, or until soft when pierced with a fork. Garnish with flax oil. Other garnishes can include chopped green onions, soy cheese, and salsa.

 *Vegetables*

Kale with Lemon   **Serves 4**

Kale is one of my favorite vegetables and it also has terrific health benefits for women since it is a good source of calcium and other essential nutrients like lutein which supports the health of your eyes.

1 bunch of kale
1 lemon, cut into quarters
Soy sauce

Rinse kale well and remove stems. Steam for 5-6 minutes or until leaves wilt and are tender. Dress lightly with soy sauce and lemon juice.

Simple Steamed Cabbage   **Serves 4**

1 small head cabbage, quartered
1 teaspoon chopped parsley
1 teaspoon olive oil
pinch of sea salt (optional)

Steam cabbage until tender. Sprinkle with olive oil and parsley.

Jessica's Favorite Broccoli   **Serves 4**

1 pound broccoli
1 tablespoons flax oil
Pinch of sea salt (optional)
Squeeze of lemon

Cut the broccoli into small flowerets; steam until tender. Squeeze lemon juice over broccoli and add the flax oil. Mix and serve.

Cauliflower with Flax Oil   Serves 4

1 medium head cauliflower
2 tablespoons flax oil
pinch of sea salt (optional)

Break the cauliflower into small flowerets. Steam until tender. Toss with flax oil and sea salt.

Roasted Rosemary Potatoes   Serves 4-6

I love roasted potatoes! This is a wonderful potato recipe that I like to make when I serve roasted chicken.

4 cups red potatoes – about 4 or 5 large red potatoes
1 tablespoon dried rosemary, crushed
3 tablespoons of olive oil
2 garlic cloves, minced
¼ teaspoon black pepper (optional)
Sea salt

Preheat oven to 400 degrees. Cut potatoes into bite size pieces and put into plastic bag. Add olive oil, rosemary, garlic, and black pepper to bag. Close bag and shake to coat all of the potato pieces.

Line a baking tray with foil and put potatoes on to tray. Arrange evenly in one layer. Sprinkle salt onto potatoes and bake for 30-35 minutes until brown and cooked through. During cooking stir the potatoes once if desired.

Honey Carrots **Serves 4**

This is one of my favorite side dishes. The warm honey brings out the natural sweetness of the carrots.

3 cups carrots, sliced thin
1 teaspoon honey
1 teaspoon almond oil
Salt (optional)

Cut carrots into thin slices and steam for 6-8 minutes, or until tender. Using the same saucepan pour out the cooking water and on low heat add the honey and oil and mix well. Add carrots and mix all ingredients together. Add a pinch of salt before serving.

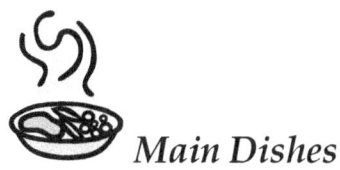 *Main Dishes*

Mega Greens Rice Bowl   **Serves 4**

This dish is a satisfying way to get a large serving of healthy greens. A delicious sauce is Organicville's Island Teriyaki (organicvillefoods.com). Their sauce is made with agave nectar instead of cane sugar.

4 cups kale, cut into bite size pieces (about ½ bunch)
3 cups baby bok choy, chopped
1 cup of white mushrooms, sliced
1 carrot, finely chopped
8 ounces of tofu, cubed
3 cups cooked brown rice - ¾ cup rice per person
Teriyaki sauce – soy sauce - gomasio

Steam the carrots for 4 minutes and then add the kale, bok choy, mushrooms, and tofu. Steam for 5 minutes. Serve in a deep bowl over rice with your choice of sauce.

Good sauces for this dish include teriyaki sauce and soy sauce. A little bit of lemon juice and gomasio also works well.

Teriyaki Tofu Wrap **Serves 2**

The tofu and teriyaki flavors blend delightfully with the vegetables. This is a light and delicious wrap.

2 brown rice tortillas
6 ounces of baked tofu, cubed or sliced (see recipe)
¼ red pepper, sliced thinly
2 radishes, sliced thinly
1 cup salad greens
½ cup sprouts
2 tablespoons teriyaki sauce

Lightly heat up the tortilla until soft. Layer the vegetables inside and top with the tofu. Lightly pour the sauce on top. Wrap and serve.

Summertime Veggie Pasta **Serves 4**

This light pasta is one of my favorite dishes to eat during the summer. The pasta and sauce are light but filling. It's a dish that I love to share to share with friends.

1 box quinoa elbow pasta (8 ounce box)
½ onion, diced
2 cans Italian seasoned diced tomatoes
1 can garbanzo beans
1 carrot, shredded
1½ cups cooked Brussels sprouts or broccoli
½ teaspoon dried basil
2 teaspoons olive oil
⅛ teaspoon pepper
Pinch of salt (optional)

Cook pasta according to package directions. In a saucepan on medium heat add olive oil and onions. Sautee until onions are translucent. Add remainder of ingredients and bring to a simmer. Cook on low heat for 10 minutes. Combine the cooked noodles with the sauce.

Eggplant Parmesan **Serves 4-6**

I love eggplant Parmesan. It is a rich and extremely delicious entree. This version, while wonderful, takes a little more time and has a few more steps than most of my entrees. Even though I use substitutions for the cheese, the dish is still very rich and I recommend saving it for a special occasion or party. You will wow your guests with how tasty it is! My favorite cheese alternative is by Follow Your Heart. Their products can be found in health food stores or at followyourheart.com

1 eggplant, cut into ⅓ - ½ inch slices (peeling is optional)
2 eggs, beaten
1 ¼ cups gluten free breadcrumbs
3 cups of pasta sauce, tomato and basil flavor
8 ounces of mozzarella cheese, shredded
⅓ cup Parmesan or soy Parmesan cheese, grated
¼ cup olive oil - divided

Arrange the eggplant slices in a colander or on a rack placed over the sink. Sprinkle all of the slices generously with salt and let stand 30 minutes; the eggplant slices will release water. Rinse and pat dry. Next, dip each slice in the beaten egg and coat with breadcrumbs.

Heat a portion of the olive oil in a skillet over medium heat. Cook the eggplant until golden on each side, about 2-3 minutes. If necessary, reduce the heat to medium-low. Repeat until all of the eggplant is cooked.

Preheat the oven 350°. Arrange half the eggplant slices on the bottom of a lightly oiled baking dish (a 9x9 or 9x12 pan works well). Spread half of the pasta sauce on top. Sprinkle with half of the mozzarella and half of the Parmesan cheese. Repeat with the next layer.

Bake 25-30 minutes or until mixture is bubbly.

Parmesan Chicken Pasta   **Serves 4**

This dish is a crowd pleaser that I often serve when I have friends over. The Parmesan cheese adds a delightful tanginess that rounds out the dish perfectly.

6 cups gluten free pasta, cooked
1 ½ cups roasted chicken, cubed
⅔ cup diced carrots
⅔ cup diced red onion
½ onion, diced
1 small tomato, finely chopped
3 cups broccoli, chopped into bite size pieces
⅔ cup chicken broth (recommended) or water
1 teaspoon dried basil
1 tablespoon olive oil
Soy Parmesan cheese or regular, grated (to taste)
Generous pinch of pepper
Salt (optional)

In a frying pan on medium heat add the olive oil. Add the onion and sauté until onion begin to turn translucent. Add all vegetables except tomatoes and cook for 1-2 minutes. Add chicken broth, chicken, tomatoes, basil, and pepper. Turn heat to low, cover and simmer for 5-7 minutes or until broth has cooked down. Add more broth if needed.

Add the sauce to the pasta. Serve with Parmesan cheese.

Turkey Bolognese   **Serves 2-4**

This dish cooks up quickly and is very satisfying. This is a versatile recipe. You can add all kinds of vegetables and it will taste great.

½ lb. ground turkey
2 cans of diced tomatoes
1 can tomato paste
½ onion, diced
1 carrot, diced
1 zucchini, diced
1 teaspoon basil
1 teaspoon oregano
1 tablespoon olive oil
¼ teaspoon salt (optional)
½ teaspoon black pepper (optional)
Water (optional)

Heat pan on medium and add olive oil. Add onion and sauté until translucent. Add turkey and all herbs and spices. Cook until turkey has browned and cooked thoroughly. Add tomatoes, tomato paste, carrots, and zucchini. Cook on low heat for 12-15 minutes. If sauce is too thick add a small amount of water until desired consistency is reached. Serve over brown rice spaghetti.

Simple Broiled Tuna   **Serves 4**

4 fillets of tuna, 4 ounces. each
2 teaspoons olive oil
Squeeze of lemon juice
pinch of sea salt

Baste the tuna fillets with oil; then sprinkle with lemon juice. Place tuna in a broiler pan. and broil until the level of doneness that you prefer (rare or well-done).

Simple Steamed Salmon   **Serves 4**

4 fillets of salmon, 4 ounces. each

* 1 cup water
Squeeze of lemon

Combine water and lemon juice in a steamer. Place salmon fillets in streamer basket. Cook to the level of doneness that you prefer.

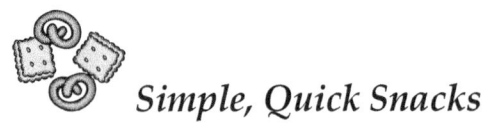 *Simple, Quick Snacks*

Trail Mix   **Makes ¾ cup**

¼ cup raw unsalted pumpkin seeds
¼ cup raw unsalted sunflower seeds
¼ cup raisins

Combine and store in a container in the refrigerator. This trail mix is very high in essential fatty acids, calcium, magnesium, and iron. I use it for a snack food to replace stressful and unhealthy sugar-based sweets seeds and chocolate. It is a great mix to take on trips, and I eat it often for breakfast.

Rice Cakes with Nut Butter and Jam   **Serves 2**

4 unsalted rice cakes
2 tablespoons raw almond butter
2 tablespoons fruit preserves (no sugar added)

Spread rice cakes with almond butter and fruit preserves for a quick snack. *Herbal tea makes a good accompaniment.*

Rice Cakes with Tuna Fish   **Serves 2**

4 unsalted rice cakes
4 ounces tuna fish
1 teaspoon low-calorie mayonnaise

Spread rice cakes with tuna fish and mayonnaise. *This is an excellent high-protein, high-carbohydrate snack.*

Apple with Almond Butter   Serves 2

1 apple, sliced
1 tablespoon raw almond butter

Spread almond butter on thin apple slices.

Banana with Sesame Butter   Serves 2

1 banana, halved
1 tablespoon raw sesame butter

Spread sesame butter on each half of a ripe banana.

7

Stress Reduction for Irregular Menstruation

Irregular and heavy menstrual bleeding seems to cause adverse emotional as well as physical symptoms in many women. Depression can accompany fatigue, and some women note a real decline in zest and energy levels. They complain that as their blood count drops or their menstrual periods become heavier and longer, their joy of living drops, too. Also, because they have less energy, many of these women find that they handle stress less effectively. Small work or family upsets that would normally seem insignificant become magnified. A woman who is tired and has little reserve because of a significant menstrual bleeding problem may find that major life stresses, such as job loss, death of a loved one, or divorce, seem impossible to deal with.

Exercises for Relaxation

To help you cope with the emotional stresses that may become magnified while you are resolving a menstrual bleeding problem, I recommend a variety of relaxation methods. Deep breathing, meditation, affirmations, and visualizations can help promote a sense of calm and well-being if practiced on a regular basis. In this chapter, I include exercises from all four categories for you to try. Pick those you enjoy most and practice them on a regular basis.

I have taught these exercises to women patients and love to practice them myself. My patients have been very enthusiastic about the results they attain practicing stress-reduction exercises. They often tell me that they feel much calmer and happier. They also find their physical health has improved. A calm mind seems to have beneficial effects on the body's physiology and chemistry, restoring the body to a normal condition.

First step: Find a comfortable position. For many women, this means lying on their back. You may also do most of the exercises sitting up. Try to keep your spine as straight as possible. Your arms and legs should be uncrossed. It is important that your clothes be loose and comfortable.

Second step: Focus your attention on the exercises; do not allow distracting thoughts to interfere with your concentration. Close your eyes and take a few deep breaths. This will help to quiet your mind and remove your thoughts from the problems and tasks of the day.

Relaxation Methods

Exercise 1: Vitality Breathing

Lie flat on your back with your knees pulled up. Keep your feet slightly apart. Breathe in and out through your nose, if possible.

Inhale deeply. As you breathe in, allow your stomach to relax so that the air flows into your abdomen. Let your stomach balloon out as you breathe in. Visualize the lowest parts of your lungs filling up with air.

Imagine that the air you are breathing in is filled with energy and vitality. Vitality is filling every cell in your body. It fills you with a sensation of warmth and healing. Now, exhale deeply. As you breathe out, imagine the air being pushed out from the bottom of your lungs to the top.

Repeat this sequence until your body feels relaxed and your breathing is slow and regular.

Exercise 2: Color Breathing

Color breathing has traditionally been used to heal the body, calm the nerves, and strengthen the body's energy field. Indian and Chinese spiritual traditions described the body's energy field in detail as far back as 3000 B.C. Intuitives in our culture are able to describe the energy field as lights or colors that emanate from the body.

Different parts of the body appear to emanate different colors: the legs emanate red; the pelvis and intestines, orange; the solar plexus, yellow; the heart, green; the throat, blue; the eyes and pituitary, violet; and the top of the head, white. According to the traditional models, each color gives energy and strength to the body part to which it corresponds. When you are calm and relaxed, the human energy field looks radiant, harmonious, and full of color. It has the soft, rounded shape of an egg.

Color breathing is a powerful technique to balance the energy field of the body and help heal the systems that are deficient, through a combination of breath work and visualization.

- Sit or lie in a comfortable position. Take a deep breath and imagine that the earth beneath you is filled with the color green. This color goes 50 feet below you into the earth. Imagine that you are opening up energy centers on the bottom of your feet.

- As you inhale, visualize the beautiful color green (like the green of a park or golf course) filling up your feet. See the bones of your feet filling with green, especially the marrow (or center of the bones) where the red cells are made. See the marrow filling with a beautiful green color.

- As you inhale, bring the color green up through the center of your leg bones, hip bones, pelvis, spine, ribs, arms, neck, and head. See it flow out of your bones and fill the air around you. Exhale the green slowly out of your lungs. Repeat this process slowly 5 times.

- Now visualize the veins and arteries of your body. They form a network of vessels linking all parts of your body by circulating the blood and oxygen.

- As you inhale, bring the color red into your blood vessels. Visualize the blood vessels in all parts of your body. The blood vessels of your legs, hips, pelvis, abdomen, chest, arms, neck, and head are filled with bright red. Exhale the red slowly out of your body. See the color fill the air around you. Repeat this process slowly 5 times.

Exercise 3: Meditation

This meditation requires you to sit quietly and engage in a simple and repetitive activity. (This can be very difficult at first.) By emptying your mind, you give yourself a rest. The metabolism of your body slows down. The brain wave slows from the fast beta wave that predominates during the normal working day to a slower alpha or theta wave. This slower pattern is what appears during sleep or in the period of deep relaxation just before falling asleep. Meditating gives the mind a vacation from tension and worry.

- Lie or sit in a very comfortable position.

- Close your eyes and breathe deeply. Let your breathing be slow and relaxed.

- Focus all your attention on your breathing. Notice the movement of your chest and abdomen in and out.

- Block out all other thoughts, feelings, and sensations. If you feel your attention wandering, bring it back to your breathing.

- Count to 1 as you inhale, 2 as you exhale, 3 as you inhale, 4 as you exhale, until you reach 20. Repeat this exercise at least 5 times. For the best results, repeat the sequence for as long as you are able, up to 5 minutes.

Exercise 4: Affirmations for Irregular and Heavy Menstrual Bleeding

The use of affirmations can be a very powerful therapeutic tool when you are embarking on a program to relieve irregular or heavy menstrual bleeding. This is because your state of health is determined by the interaction between your mind and body. You are constantly sending yourself messages – thousands each day – that have a profound effect on your body chemistry and physiology.

I emphasize to all my patients that the body and mind must work together in a positive way for optimal healing to take place. For example, if a patient who has come to me for a weight-loss program has a poor self-image, she will constantly be criticizing herself for the way she looks. This will be reflected in her countenance, posture, mood, and even her ability to follow a beneficial and healthful weight-loss regimen.

The following exercise will help you reprogram yourself toward restoring a more healthy menstrual cycle. Sit in a comfortable position. Repeat the following affirmations three times. Be sure to do an exercise when you are feeling calm and receptive.

- My body is able to regulate its menstrual bleeding pattern.

- I have the perfect amount of menstrual bleeding each month.

- I lose the right amount of blood each month to keep my body healthy.

- I never spot between menstrual cycles.

- I am blood-clot free.

- I have a moderate, comfortable menstrual flow.

- My menstrual cycle comes at the right time each month; I have a regular cycle.

- My ovaries and uterus are healthy.

- My thyroid is healthy and helps regulate my menstrual flow.

- I enjoy my menstrual cycle.

- I eat the food that helps regulate my menstrual flow.

- My body desires food that is high in essential nutrients, vitamins, and minerals.

- I take time each day to relax and enjoy myself.

- I practice the stress-reduction techniques that keep me calm and peaceful.

- I exercise on a regular basis. I do the exercises that I need for a healthy female reproductive tract.

- I create perfect health and well-being within my body.

Exercise 5: Visualization for Irregular and Heavy Menstrual Bleeding

Visualization exercises provide a technique for imagining your body the way you want it to be. This is a very powerful therapeutic tool that I have been using for many years with patients. The technique was pioneered by Carl Simonton, M.D., a cancer radiation therapist, who used this technique with his patients and described the results in his book *Getting Well Again*. He had his patients see their cancers as being small and weak and their immune systems as being big, strong, and capable of destroying the puny cancers (instead of the other way around). He saw many patients go into remission as they visualized their immune systems becoming healthy, using a variety of powerful images such as knights on white horses and jet planes. Visualization exercises can actually let you use imagery to lay down a mental blueprint for a healthier body.

- Close your eyes. Begin to breathe deeply. Inhale and let the air out slowly. Feel your body begin to relax. Imagine that you can look inside your uterus.

- See the lining of your uterus. It is a lush, blood-rich cushion of tissue.

- Imagine that your uterus is currently in the state that occurs right before your menstrual cycle begins. The blood vessels in the lining of the uterus begin to constrict. See them become coiled and narrow. Visualize them as they begin to release the perfect amount of blood from the uterine lining.

- The blood flows out of the uterus in a moderate, regular flow. See the blood leave the uterus in a steady, healthy manner.

- See the uterine lining slough off into the blood flow so that the uterus can prepare for the next month's cycle.

- Visualize your ovaries and tubes as they connect into the sides of the uterus. Your ovaries are shaped like almonds. They are pink and healthy looking. See them put out healthy levels of your female hormones, estrogen and progesterone. Your ovaries are perfectly regulated and function well each month.

- See the hormones leaving the ovaries to regulate your menstrual flow.

- Now stop visualizing the scene and go back to deep breathing.

- Open your eyes and feel very good.

Putting Your Stress Management Program Together

This chapter has introduced many different ways to help you handle stress better, as well as exercises for improved mind-body health. This can be very useful while you are in the healing stages of irregular and heavy menstrual bleeding. Try each exercise at least once. Experiment with them until you find the combination that works for you. Doing all seven will take no longer than 20 to 30 minutes, depending on how much time you wish to spend with each one. Ideally, the exercises should be done on a daily basis for at least a few minutes each day. Over time, they will help you gain insight into your negative beliefs and change them into positive new ones. Your ability to cope with stress should be tremendously improved.

8

Exercises for Irregular Menstruation

Women who have a problem with irregular and heavy menstrual bleeding tend to be very tired; they often find that moderate to brisk exercise is difficult for them because they lack stamina and endurance. The fatigue problem tends to resolve as the anemia and bleeding are corrected nutritionally. In the meantime, women with these conditions may completely stop a regular exercise program in an attempt to avoid feeling tired.

However, complete avoidance of exercise is not healthy, for it reduces oxygenation and circulation to vital organs, such as the brain and heart, as well as all the cells of the body. Gentle exercise such as deep breathing exercises, progressive muscle relaxation, range-of-motion exercises to keep the joints mobile, and slow relaxed walking promote good oxygenation and circulation and can even help to increase energy. The key is to exercise in a gentle, slow fashion.

I have included in this chapter several general fitness and flexibility exercises you can use to promote health and well-being. You may want to combine them with gentle aerobic exercise like walking. You can also combine them with the stretches and acupressure points described in Chapters 10 and 11.

Exercise Techniques

Exercise 1: Deep Breathing

Deep, slow abdominal breathing is essential for women with fibroids. It expands your lungs and allows you to bring adequate oxygen, the fuel for metabolic activity, to all the tissues of your body. Deep breathing will relax tight and contracted pelvic, abdominal, and low back muscles, thereby helping to relieve menstrual pain and distress. It also helps to relax the entire body and strengthens the muscles in the chest and abdomen. Deep breathing helps to stabilize mood and reduce both depression and anxiety, so it is very important for emotional well-being. In contrast, rapid, shallow breathing decreases your oxygen supply, which builds up lactic acid in the pelvic muscles, keeping them tense and tight.

Lie flat on your back with your knees pulled up. Keep your feet slightly apart. Try to breathe in and out through your nose.

Inhale deeply. As you breathe in, allow your stomach to relax so that the air flows into your abdomen. Your stomach should balloon out as you breathe in. Visualize your lungs filling up with air so that your chest swells out.

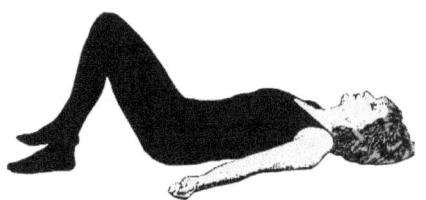

Imagine that the air you breathe is filling your body with energy

Exhale deeply. As you breathe out, let your stomach and chest collapse. Imagine the air being pushed out, first from your abdomen and then from your lungs.

Exercise 2: Progressive Muscle Relaxation

Women who are anemic due to irregular and heavy menstruation may have muscles that are tense and tight because of inadequate oxygenation and blood flow. Lactic acid tends to accumulate in these muscles, and muscle tension can become a chronic problem. Movement effectively breaks up this pattern of chronically tight muscles. Unfortunately, women with anemia tend to become less active as their fatigue worsens. While strenuous exercise may be too difficult for a woman with anemia, it is still very important to keep the muscles loose and limber. Besides feeling more relaxed, supple muscles have a beneficial effect on mood and induce a sense of peace and calm. The following exercise will aid in releasing muscle tension.

Lie in a comfortable position. Allow your arms to rest limply, palms down. Practice your deep abdominal breathing as you do this exercise. Clench your hands into fists and hold them tightly for 15 seconds. As you do this, relax the rest of your body. Then let your hands relax.

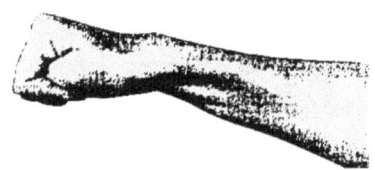

Now, tense and relax the following parts of your body in this order: face, shoulders, back, stomach, pelvis, legs, feet, and toes. Hold each part tensed for 15 seconds and then relax your body for 30 seconds before going on to the next part.

Visualize the tense part contracting, becoming tighter and tighter. On relaxing, see the energy flowing into the entire body like a gentle wave, making all the muscles soft and pliable. Finish the exercise by shaking your hands. Imagine the remaining tension flowing out of your fingertips.

Exercise 3: Joint Flexibility

It is very important that women with irregular and heavy menstrual bleeding maintain full range of motion and flexibility in all the joints of the body to reduce the tendency of muscle tension. The following exercise helps to stretch and release tension in the muscles around the joints. This exercise is similar to the "range-of-motion" sequence that physicians may use when testing a patient for joint limitations such as arthritis produces. The exercises are also thought to stimulate the acupuncture meridians as based on the work of Motoyama, a Japanese researcher. In his book, *Theories of the Chakras: Bridge to Higher Consciousness*, Motoyama discusses the importance of these exercises in opening the acupuncture meridians.

Sit on the floor with your legs stretched out in front. Place your hands at your sides.

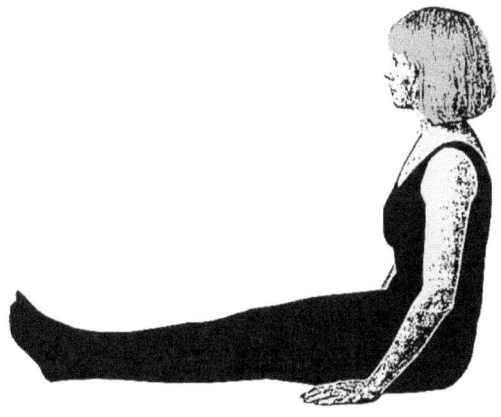

Toes: Slowly flex and extend the toes without moving your feet or ankles. Repeat 10 times.

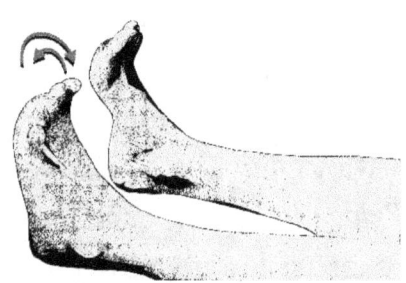

Ankles: Slowly flex and extend the ankle joints. Repeat 10 times. Separate your legs slightly, then rotate your ankles in each direction 10 times. Be sure to keep your heels on the floor.

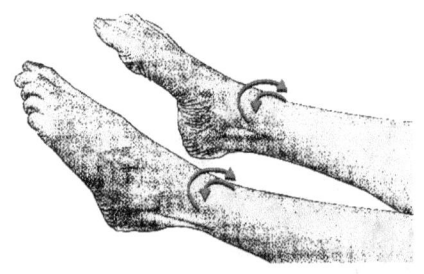

Knees: Still resting in the sitting position, bend the right leg at the knee, bringing the heel near the right buttock. Then lift the right leg off the floor, straightening the right knee. Repeat 10 times. Then do the same exercise with the left leg.

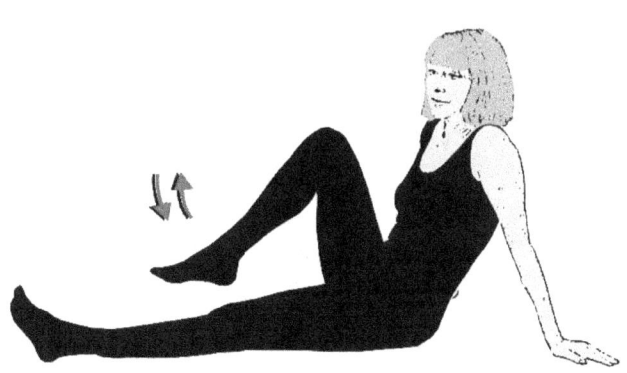

Hold the thigh near the chest with both hands. Rotate your lower leg in a circular motion about the knee 10 times clockwise and then 10 times counterclockwise. Repeat with the left leg.

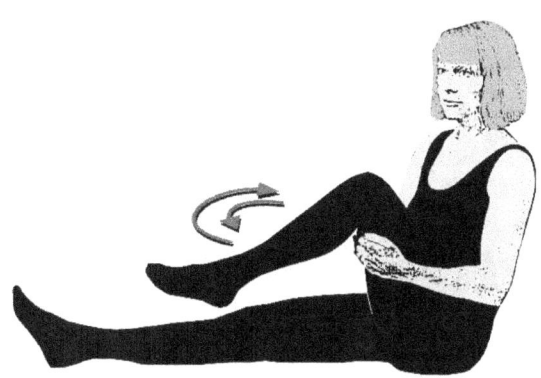

Hips: Bend the right leg so that you can place your right foot on the left thigh. Hold the right knee with the right hand and hold the right ankle with the left hand. Then gently move the right knee up and down with the right hand. Repeat with the left leg.

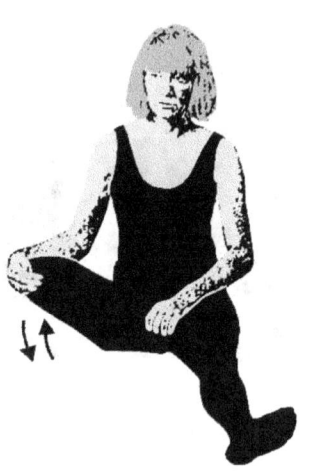

While you are sitting in the same position, rotate the right knee clockwise 10 times and then counterclockwise 10 times. This improves the flexibility of the hip joints. Repeat on the left side.

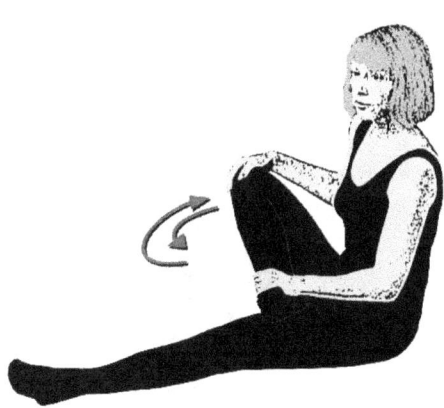

While sitting, bring the soles of the feet together, bringing the heels close to the body. Gently push the knees to the floor and then let them come up again. Repeat 10 times.

Fingers: Sit on the floor with your legs stretched out in front of you. Lift your arms up to shoulder height, keeping them straight. Open your hands wide. Flex the fingers, closing them over the thumbs to make a fist. Repeat 10 times.

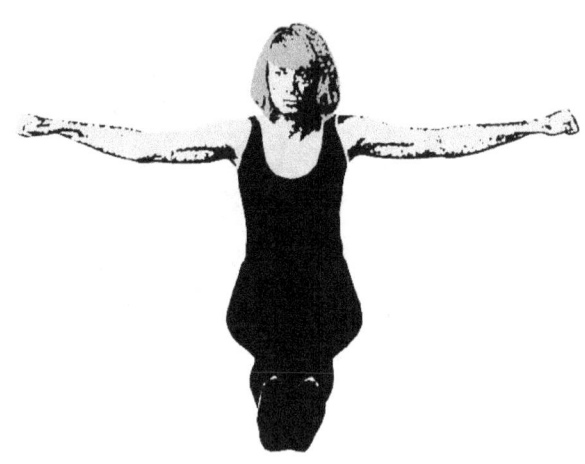

Wrists: Flex and extend your wrists. Repeat 10 times.

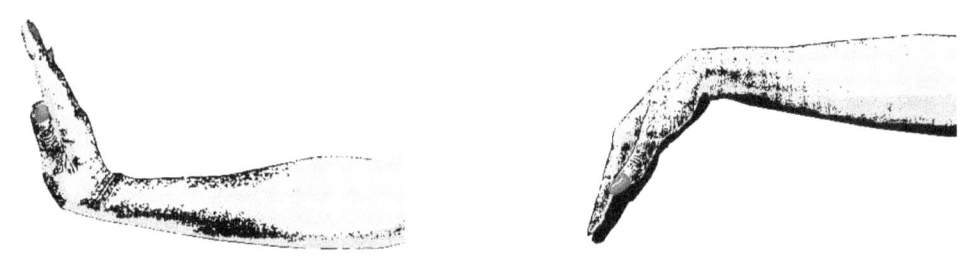

Sitting in the same position, rotate your wrists clockwise and counter-clockwise. Repeat 10 times.

Sitting in the same position, hold your hands in extension and move each hand from side to side at the wrist. Repeat 10 times.

Elbows: Remaining in the same position, stretch out your arms at shoulder height with the palms facing upward. Then bend your arms at the elbow so that your fingers touch the shoulders, and straighten out your arms again. Repeat 10 times with arms extended sideways and ten times with arms facing forward.

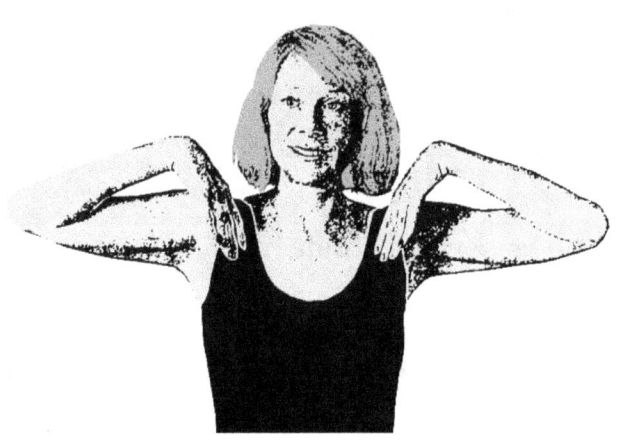

Shoulders: From the same sitting position, with your arms bent and fingertips touching the shoulders, make a circular motion with your elbows. Repeat 10 times clockwise and 10 times counterclockwise.

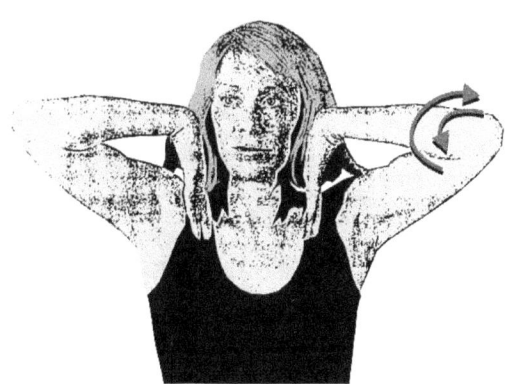

Spine: Remain sitting with your legs together straight out in front of you. Reach over and touch your legs or, without straining, your toes without bending your knees. Repeat 10 times.

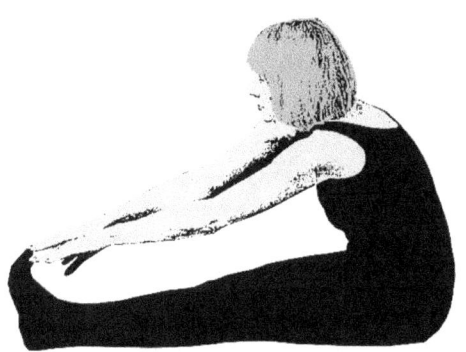

Waist: Stand up and slowly reach over and touch your lower legs or, without straining, your toes as you bend at the waist. Try to keep your knees straight. Repeat 10 times. If you have lower back problems do these two positions with caution.

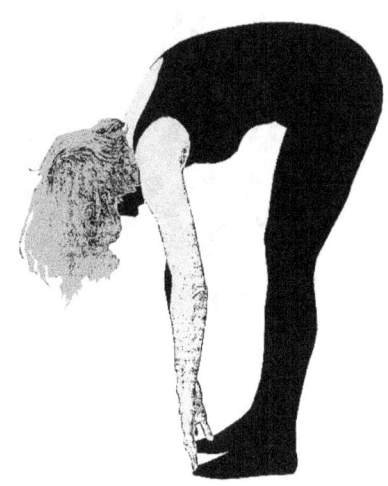

9

Stretches for Irregular Menstruation

In this chapter I present a series of specific stretches that will gently stretch every muscle in your body and will energize and balance the female reproductive tract, breasts, thyroid, and endocrine system. These poses also help optimize the health and well-being of the digestive tract, nervous system, circulation, and all other organ systems of the body. For those women whose anemia is due to irregular and heavy menstrual bleeding, these poses will provide the benefits of promoting oxygenation and better circulation to the pelvic area. This can have a beneficial effect on menstrual function. The poses will also help reduce muscle tension in the pelvic area. An added benefit for women who are fatigued, due to anemia, can be an increase in vigor and stamina. I do stretches frequently as part of my own exercise routine.

General Techniques for Stretches

When doing stretches, it is important that you focus and concentrate on the positions. First, let your mind visualize how the exercise is to look, and then follow with the correct body placement in the pose. The exercises are done through slow, controlled stretching movements. This slowness allows you to have greater control over your body movements. You minimize the possibility of injury and maximize the benefit to the particular part of the body to which your attention is being directed.

Pay close attention to the initial instructions when beginning an exercise. Look at the placement of the body as shown in the photographs. This is very important, for if the pose is practiced properly, you are much more likely to have relief of your symptoms.

Remember the following as you begin these exercises:

- Try to visualize the pose in your mind, then follow with proper placement of the body

- Move slowly through the pose. This will help promote flexibility of the muscles and prevent injury

- Follow the breathing instructions provided in the exercise. Most important, do not hold your breath. Allow your breath to flow in and out easily and effortlessly.

If you practice these stretches regularly in a slow, unhurried fashion, you will gradually loosen your muscles, ligaments, and joints. You may be surprised at how supple you can become over time. If you experience any pain or discomfort, you have probably overreached your current ability and should immediately reduce the amount of the stretching until you can proceed without discomfort. Be careful, as muscular injuries can take quite a while to heal. If you do strain a muscle, I have found that immediately applying ice to the injured area for 10 minutes is quite helpful. Continue to use the ice pack two to three times a day for several days. If the pain persists, see your doctor immediately.

Stretching Techniques

Stretch 1

This exercise improves blood circulation through the pelvis and thereby stabilizes menstrual function. It helps to calm anxiety and also strengthens the back and abdominal muscles.

Lie down and press the small of your back into the floor. This permits you to use your abdominal muscles without straining your lower back.

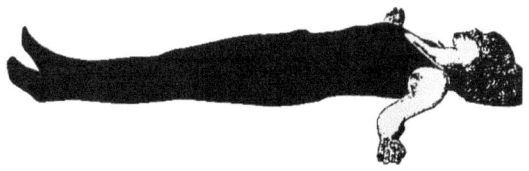

Raise your right leg slowly while breathing in. Keep your back flat on the floor and let the rest of your body remain relaxed. Move your leg very slowly; imagine your leg being pulled up smoothly by a spring. Do not move your leg in a jerky manner. Hold for a few breaths. Lower your leg and breathe out.

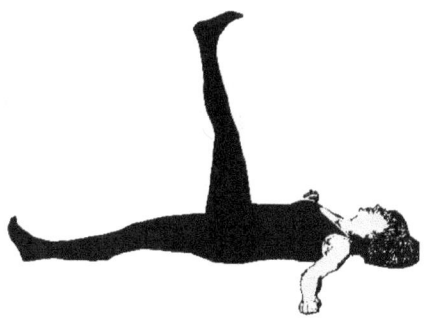

Repeat the same exercise with your left leg. Then alternate legs, repeating the exercise 5 to 10 times.

Stretch 2

This exercise energizes and rejuvenates the female reproductive tract and tones the abdominal organs (pancreas, liver, and adrenals). It emphasizes freer pelvic movement with controlled breathing.

Lie on your back with your knees bent and your feet on the floor close to your buttocks.

Exhale and press the lower back into the floor, raising the buttocks slightly

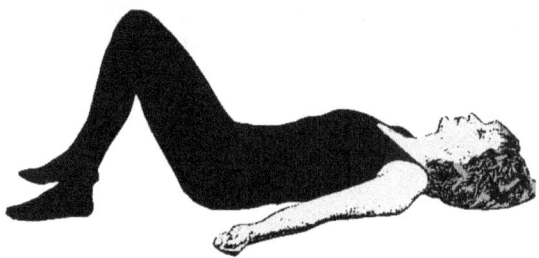

Arch the back slightly. Inhale and lift your lower back off the floor. This stretches the region from the sternum to the pelvis.

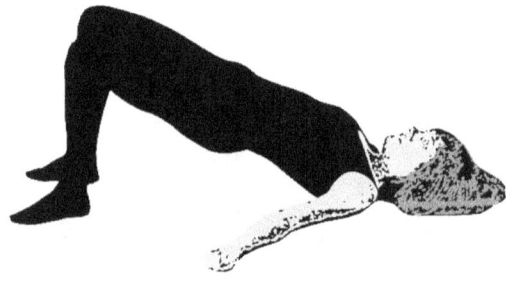

Repeat this exercise 10 times. Always lift your navel up on the in-breath. Always elongate your spine and press the lower back down on the out-breath.

Stretch 3

This exercise energizes the entire female reproductive tract, thyroid, liver, intestines, and kidneys. It may be helpful for women with anemia due to dysfunctional bleeding by improving circulation and oxygenation to the pelvic region. This exercise also strengthens the lower back, abdomen, buttocks, and legs, and prevents lower back pain and cramps.

Lie face down on the floor. Make fists with both your hands and place them under your hips. This prevents compression of the lumbar spine while doing the exercise.

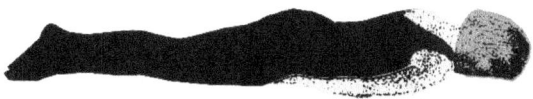

Straighten your body and raise your right leg with an upward thrust as high as you can, keeping your hips on your fists. Hold for 5 to 20 seconds if possible.

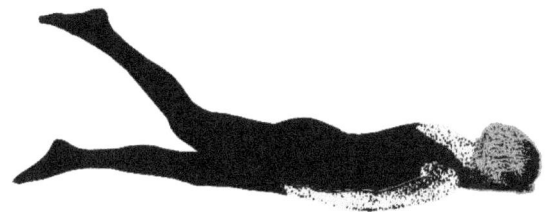

Lower the leg and slowly return to your original position. Repeat with the left leg, then with both legs together. Remember to keep your hips resting on your fists. Repeat 10 times.

Stretch 4

This exercise helps to relieve anemia-related fatigue and lack of vitality due to irregular and heavy menstruation, elevating your mood and improving stamina. This exercise also stretches the entire spine and helps to relieve lower back pain and cramps. It stretches the abdominal muscles and strengthens the back, hips, and thighs. It also stimulates the digestive organs and endocrine glands.

Lie face down on the floor, arms at your sides.

Slowly bend your legs at the knees and bring your feet up toward your buttocks.

Reach back with your arms and carefully take hold of first one foot and then the other. Flex your feet to make grasping them easier.

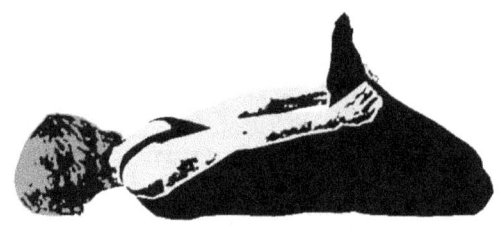

Inhale and raise your trunk from the floor as far as possible and lift your head. Bring your knees as close together as possible.

Squeeze the buttocks while raising them off the floor. Imagine your body looking like a gently curved bow. Hold for 10 to 15 seconds.

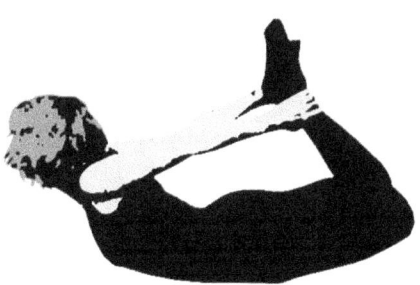

Slowly release the posture. Allow your chin to touch the floor and finally release your feet and return them slowly to the floor. Return to your original position. Repeat 5 times.

Stretch 5

This exercise opens the entire pelvic region and energizes the female reproductive tract. It is helpful for varicose veins and improves circulation in the legs.

Lie on your back with your legs against the wall, extended out in a V or an arc, and your arms extended to the sides.

Hips should be as close to the wall as possible, spread legs apart as far as you can while still remaining comfortable.

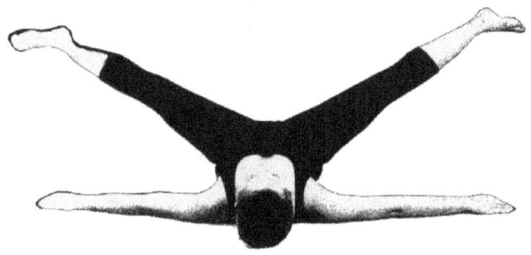

Breathing easily, hold for 1 minute, allowing the inner thighs to relax. Bring legs together and hold for 1 minute.

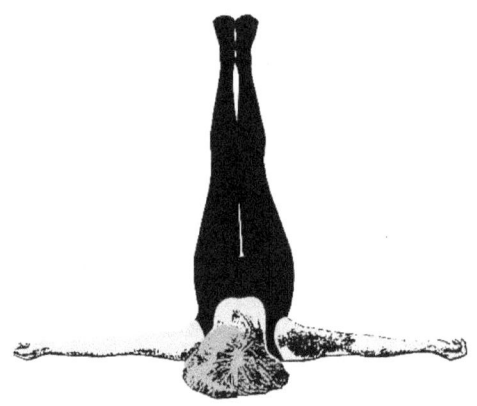

10

Acupressure for Irregular Menstruation

Acupressure is an easy-to-use method of applying finger pressure to specific points on the body in order to help prevent disease and illness. It has been an important part of traditional Chinese healing for many centuries and is often used along with herbs to promote healing.

Acupressure is based on the belief that there exists within the body a life energy or "biofield". This life energy is called chi. It is different from, yet similar to, electromagnetic energy. Health is thought to be a state in which the chi is equally distributed throughout the body and is present in sufficient amounts. It is thought to energize all the cells and tissues of the body.

The life energy is thought to run through the body in channels called meridians. When working in a healthy manner, these channels distribute the energy evenly throughout the body, sometimes on the surface of the skin and at times deep inside the body, in the organs. Disease occurs when the energy flow in a meridian is blocked or stopped. As a result, the internal organs that correspond to the meridians can show symptoms of disease. The meridian flow can be corrected by stimulating the points on the skin surface. These points can be treated easily by hand massage. When the normal flow of energy through the body is resumed, the body is believed to heal itself spontaneously.

Stimulation of the acupressure points through finger pressure can be done by you or by a friend following simple instructions. It is safe, painless, and does not require the use of needles. It can be used without the years of specialized training needed for insertion of acupuncture needles.

How to Perform Acupressure

- Acupressure may be done either by yourself or by a friend when you are relaxed. Your room should be warm and quiet. Hands should be clean and nails trimmed to avoid bruising. If your hands are cold, warm them in water.

- Choose the side of the body to work on that has the most discomfort. If both sides are equally uncomfortable, choose whichever one you want. Working on one side seems to relieve the symptoms on both sides. There appears to be a transfer of energy or information from one side to the other.

- Hold each point indicated in the exercise with a steady pressure for 1 to 3 minutes. Pressure should be applied slowly with the tips or balls of the fingers. It is best to place several fingers over the area of the point. If you feel resistance or tension in the area on which you are applying pressure, you may want to push a little harder. However, if your hand starts to feel tense or tired, lighten the pressure a bit. Make sure that your hand is comfortable. The acupressure point may feel somewhat tender. This means that the energy pathway or meridian is blocked.

- During the treatment, the tenderness in the point should slowly go away. You may also have a subjective feeling of energy radiating from this point into the body. Many patients describe this sensation as very pleasant. Don't worry if you don't feel it—not everyone does. The main goal is relief from your symptoms.

- Breathe gently while doing each exercise.

- The point that you are to hold is shown in the photograph accompanying the exercise. All these points correspond to specific points on the acupressure meridians.

- Massage the points once a day or more during the time that you have symptoms.

Acupressure Exercises

Exercise 1: Balances the Reproductive System

This exercise normalizes the energy of the reproductive organs by balancing points on the bladder meridian. It also relieves lower back pain and can help to relieve excessive menstrual bleeding.

Sit on the floor and prop your back against a wall or a heavy piece of furniture. Hold each step for 1 to 3 minutes.

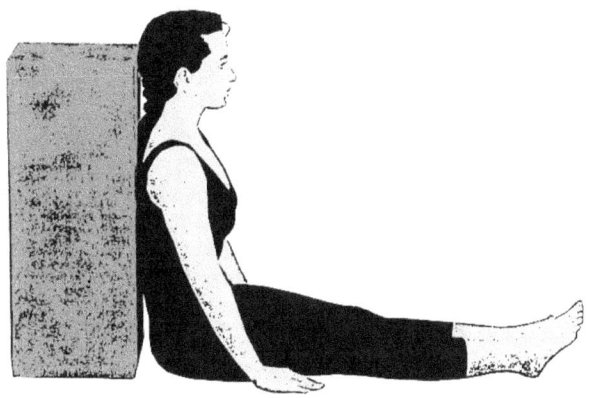

Alternative method: Lie on the floor and put your lower legs over the seat of a chair. Follow the exercise from that position.

Place left hand 1 inch above the waist on the muscle to the left side of the spine (muscle will feel firm and ropelike). Place right hand behind crease of the left knee.

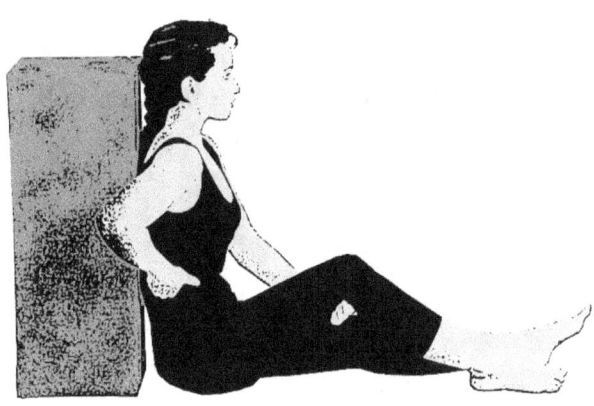

Left hand stays in the same position. Right hand is placed on the center of the back of the left calf. This is just below the fullest part of the calf.

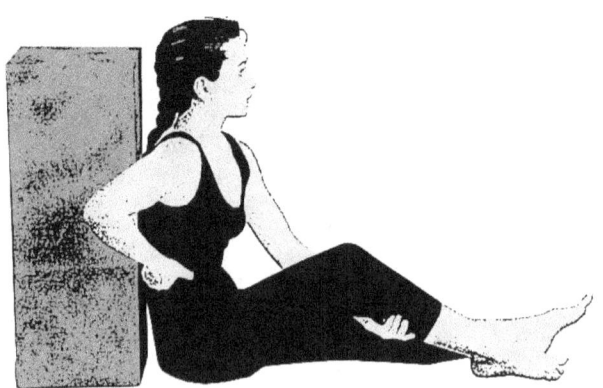

Left hand remains 1 inch above the waist on the muscle to the side of the spine. Right hand is placed just below the ankle bone on the outside of the left heel.

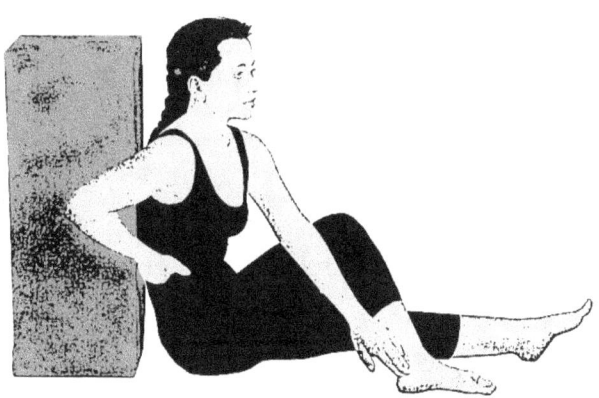

Left hand remains 1 inch above the waist on the muscle to the side of the spine. Right hand holds the front and back of the left little toe at the nail.

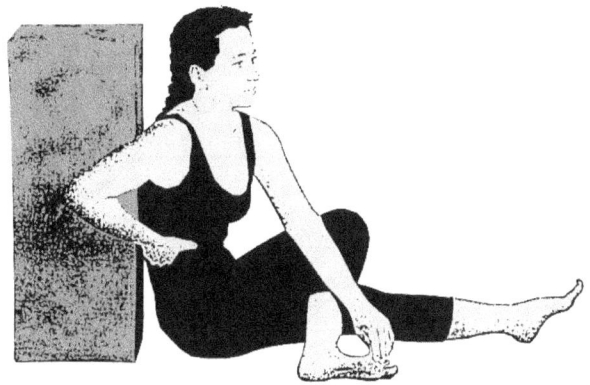

Exercise 2: Relieves Excessive Menstrual Bleeding

This exercise has been used traditionally in controlling excessive uterine bleeding.

Sit upright on a chair. Hold each step for 1 to 3 minutes.

Bend over at the waist with left hand holding point in front of ankle bone. Move hand slowly along points on leg.

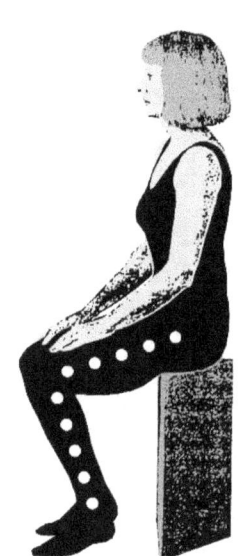 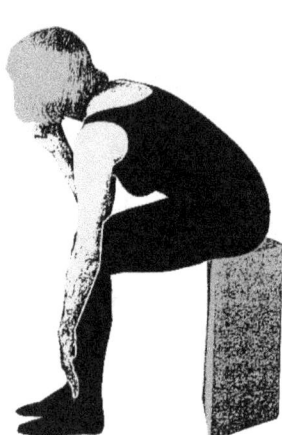

Move left hand slowly on points to the top of the thigh. Repeat on the right side with right hand.

Right hand in middle of thigh points up to groin. Repeat on other side with left hand. Circle area around navel in counterclockwise direction.

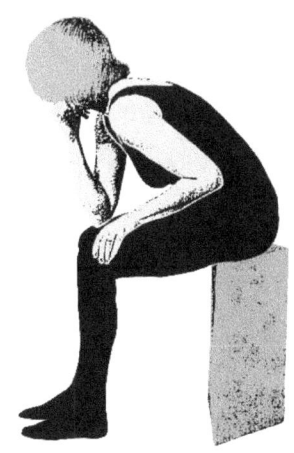 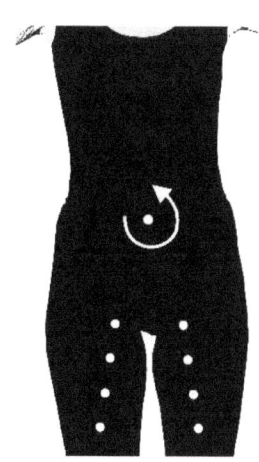

Exercise 3: Relieves Thyroid Imbalance

This exercise energizes the thyroid, which can cause excessive menstrual bleeding.

Sit upright on a chair. Hold each step for 1 to 3 minutes.

Wrap hands around shoulders with thumbs pressing gently into both sides on top of collarbone.

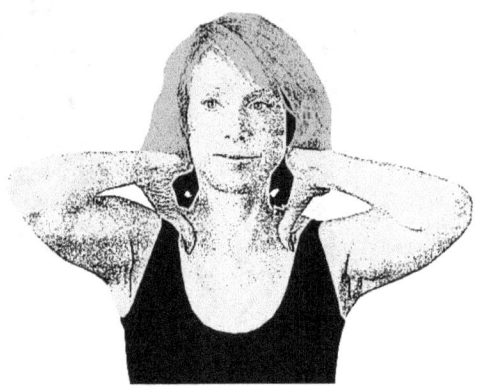

Fingers are in back and press against upper shoulders and shoulder blade area.

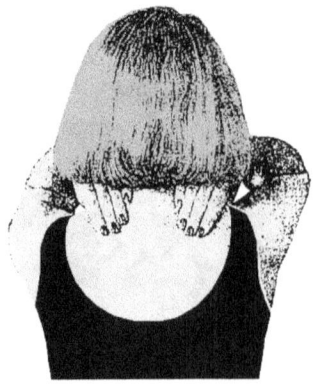

Exercise 4: Use for Relief of Anemia due to Irregular and Heavy Menstruation

This sequence of points is important for the treatment of anemia. It involves the stimulation of points on the spleen meridian that affect blood formation and menstrual problems.

Sit upright on a chair. Hold each step for 1 to 3 minutes. Right hand holds point four finger-widths above the ankle bone.

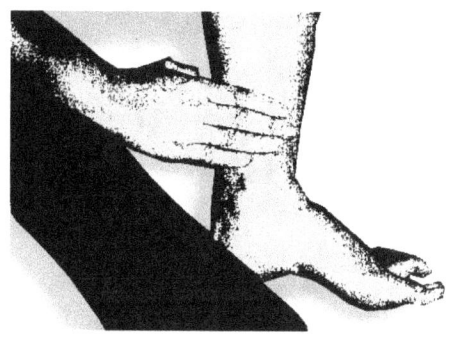

Right hand holds point above and below the nail of the big toe.

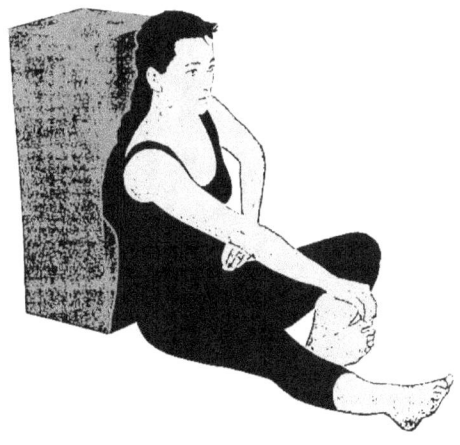

Exercise 5: Use for Relief of Fatigue and Tiredness

This exercise helps to relieve the fatigue and tiredness that commonly accompany irregular and heavy menstrual bleeding.

Sit upright on a chair. Hold each step for 1 to 3 minutes. Right hand holds a point directly between the eyebrows, where the bridge of the nose meets the forehead.

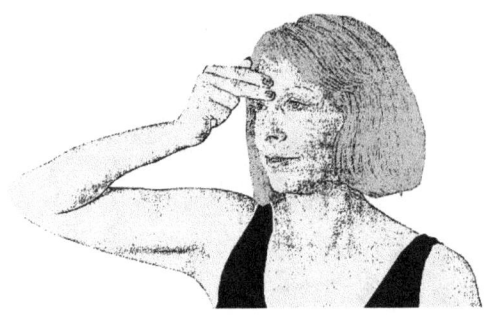

Fingers hold a point below the navel. Measure three finger-widths below the navel to find this point.

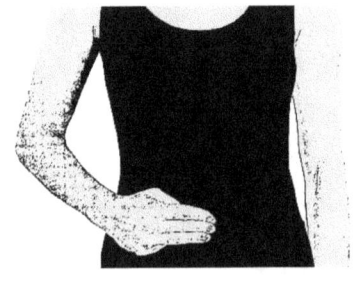

11

Drugs for Relief of Irregular Menstruation

Drugs and hormonal therapies have been the mainstay of Western medical response to excessive menstrual bleeding for the past thirty to forty years. Progestins and birth control pills have been the traditional drug treatments for this problem. Other medications, specifically the prescription antiprostaglandins, synthetic male hormones, and GnRH analogs, have been available for use in treating excessive menstrual bleeding for the past fifteen years. These more recent drug therapies have provided women with a major source of symptom relief and are still commonly used today. Women with heavy menstrual flow due to thyroid imbalance can be treated with hormone replacement therapy. All of these drugs are discussed in detail in this chapter.

Progesterone Therapy

Women who are transitioning into menopause are at high risk for heavy, irregular menstrual bleeding. This is due to the hormonal imbalance that accompanies this transition. High to normal estrogen levels with inadequate to absent progesterone levels are commonly seen in women in their forties and early fifties. Unfortunately, women in transition are usually not ideal candidates for hormone replacement therapy (HRT). HRT consists of daily administration of both estrogen and progesterone. This is because your body is producing hormones erratically, often manufacturing large amounts of estrogen. Although you are still having periods and bleeding profusely, there is plenty of estrogenic stimulation. What women don't need during this time is more estrogen.

If you are not ovulating regularly and your progesterone levels are inadequate, progesterone therapy may be the ideal treatment. In fact, progesterone—usually the synthetic progestin Provera—is the most effective medical treatment available for women in menopause transition.

Progesterone is usually prescribed alone for one week or 10 to 12 days a month in doses ranging from 5 to 10 mg per day.

Progesterone helps prevent erratic, heavy periods by making sure that any buildup of endometrial lining is completely shed each month. By promoting a regular menstrual period each month, the use of progesterone can also help reduce the number of endometrial biopsies your physician needs to perform. Eventually, estrogen levels will diminish to the point that menstruation no longer occurs. At this point, regular HRT can start. Unfortunately, progestins are not without side effects, including fatigue or depression, breast tenderness, and headaches.

Natural progesterone (made from soybeans and wild yams) is available as a skin cream or in oral micronized progesterone tablets. Natural progesterone, like the synthetic forms, can be used to oppose the high estrogen levels present at this time. The cream can be rubbed directly into the skin in areas like the abdomen, while the tablets are taken by mouth. It is worth exploring if you find that you do not tolerate the synthetic progestins well, since natural progesterone tends to cause fewer side effects. Dosage is 1/4 to 1/2 teaspoon of the cream twice daily or 50 to 200 mg of the oral tablet 10 to 12 days per month.

Low-Dose Birth Control Pills

Oral contraceptive agents are also occasionally prescribed for women in transition who are experiencing heavy menstrual flow as well as for women with pain, bleeding, or spotting due to endometriosis. The FDA now considers low-dose birth control pills safe for use by women up to age fifty, providing they are nonsmokers and do not have a history of blood clotting problems, gallbladder disease, or hypertension. There are benefits to this therapeutic approach. The low-dose pills shut down your system, replacing the high, erratic levels of hormones your body is producing with a premeasured outside source. This helps control heavy, irregular bleeding and may decrease PMS symptoms in some women. It also confers protection against unwanted pregnancy as women enter mid-life.

If the birth control pill is well matched to your body's need, your symptoms may smooth out and disappear. Unfortunately, many women can't tolerate the low-dose birth control pills. PMS-like symptoms may worsen, such as mood swings, bloating and cramps. These formulations do contain a synthetic estrogen that is much stronger than the "natural" estrogen used in HRT, such as Premarin. As a result, women on low-dose birth control pills may have an increased risk of having a stroke, developing hypertension or blood-clotting problems. However, if you have had a good experience using birth control pills in the past, you may want to explore this option.

Prostaglandin Inhibitors

These drugs, also called non-steroidal anti-inflammatory agents, are a relatively new class of prescription drugs. There is evidence that certain types of prostaglandins, specifically prostaglandin E compounds, are elevated in women with heavy menstrual bleeding. While these drugs are commonly used to treat menstrual cramps, as well as the pain and cramps caused by endometriosis, these may also be useful in reducing menstrual flow. They do this by inhibiting prostaglandin production. Mefanamic acid taken in dosages of 250 to 500 mg three times a day, or other similar anti-prostaglandin drugs may cut down on blood loss.

These medications are particularly useful for pain and bleeding problems due to endometriosis as well as the painful spasms related to menstrual cramps, since they have both anti-inflammatory and pain-killing activity. These drugs were originally developed for the treatment of arthritis and are primarily available by prescription. They include Motrin™, Naprosyn™, Anaprox™, and Ponstel™. Ibuprofen (Advil™, Nuprin™) is available in higher dosage levels as Motrin™. These drugs must be used carefully, however, since they can cause gastrointestinal bleeding and peptic ulcer disease or even reactivate a pre-existing ulcer. Approximately ten percent of women who use these medications report digestive symptoms. Heartburn, nausea, vomiting, diarrhea, constipation, and poor digestion can occur as the result of using these medications. To lessen the likelihood of these side effects, only use these medications with food and report any significant digestive symptoms to your physician. Some women report other unpleasant symptoms when using prostaglandin inhibitors like drowsiness, headaches, vertigo, dizziness, rashes, blurred vision, anemia, edema, and heart palpitations. Avoid using these drugs with aspirin, since both can cause gastrointestinal bleeding and irritation.

Danazol™

This is one of the most popular current hormonal therapies for endometriosis and is quite useful in reducing pain, bleeding, spotting, and other symptoms due to this condition. It also been used to treat fibrocystic breast disease although it has not been found to be particularly useful for fibroids. Danazol™ is marketed as Danocrine in the United States. Danazol™ is a synthetic hormone derived from the male hormone testosterone. It acts to induce a pseudo-menopause by directly depressing the output of FSH (follicle stimulating hormone) and LH (luteinizing hormone) from the pituitary and hypothalamus and lowering estrogen production by the ovaries. Because of this effect on the endocrine glands, Danazol™ is called a gonadotropin inhibitor. It also acts to alter the metabolism of estrogen and progesterone and to block the estrogen and progesterone receptors in the endometrial implants.

These changes lead to both relief of endometriosis symptoms and shrinkage of the implants. Large masses and adhesions or scar tissue actually disappear. This offers tremendous benefit to women with endometriosis, 85 percent of whom report significant relief. Danazol™ may cause the regression of fibrocystic breast lesions and can be beneficial in treating this disease.

Treatment is generally instituted for six to twelve months, depending on the severity of the disease. Danazol™ is generally prescribed in doses between 400 mg. and 800 mg., often in two divided doses. One dose is taken at night and one during the day. The drug generally reduces estrogen levels low enough to stop menstruation. This may take several months to occur and many women notice light menstrual bleeding for the first few months.

Danazol™ does have drawbacks, however. It does not cure endometriosis. One survey of 180 women conducted by the Endometriosis Association in Milwaukee, Wisconsin reported that more than 50 percent of women surveyed who had taken Danazol™ either stated they had no symptom relief or had a recurrence of symptoms immediately after stopping the drug. In other reports, twenty percent noted a recurrence of endometrial symptoms within a year after stopping Danazol™ therapy. This incidence continues to increase with time.

Another problem that many women using Danazol™ encounter is unpleasant side effects. While Danazol™ itself does not cause masculine-ization, it decreases estrogen levels significantly enough that a woman's natural male hormonal response is accentuated. This can lead to acne, abnormal hair growth, increased oiliness of the skin or hair, weight gain, decrease in breast size, deepening of the voice, and even, though rarely, clitoral hypertrophy. These masculinizing effects are, unfortunately, not always reversible.

Due to the decline in the estrogen levels, women on Danazol™ may also have menopause symptoms such as hot flashes, night sweats, and vaginal dryness. Other unpleasant side effects include bloating, fluid retention, weight gain, changes in liver function, muscle cramps, headaches, dizzy-ness, depression, and anxiety. Danazol™, for all its benefits, must be carefully monitored by a physician during the course of therapy.

GnRH Analogs (Gonadotropin-releasing hormone analogs)

Drugs such as Lupron™ and Nafarelin™ have been tested experimentally in recent years as another treatment for both fibroids and endometriosis. Since heavy menstrual bleeding is the most common symptom that women with fibroids experience, these medications may be very helpful in providing significant relief. They are chemically similar to the gonado-tropin-releasing hormone (GnRH or LH-RH) which triggers secretion of LH and FSH by the pituitary. The pituitary in turn regulates the ovarian output of estrogen and progesterone. Analog drugs are given by nasal spray or injection and, like Danazol™, inhibit the hypothalamus-pituitary-ovarian feedback loop. As a result, FSH and LH secretion is inhibited and estrogen levels decrease. Also like Danazol™, these drugs shrink endometrial implants and fibroids and are also used for the treatment of other diseases when suppression of estrogen is important, such as ovarian cysts.

One benefit of the GnRH analogs is that they don't have masculinizing side effects like Danazol™. They do, however, produce the typical symptoms of menopause—hot flashes, mood swings, back and muscle pain, and headaches. They also increase the long-term risk of osteoporosis by lowering the estrogen level and increasing calcium excretion from the body. The side effects can be quite unpleasant—I have had a number of younger women see me in consultation purely to work with the menopausal side effects that the analogs cause.

Thyroid Replacement Therapy

One common cause of heavy menstrual bleeding is low thyroid function. Hypothyroidism is easily treatable with thyroid replacement therapy. Besides correcting excessive menstrual bleeding, it corrects other common symptoms of thyroid deficiency, including constipation, skin and hair changes, weight gain, fatigue, and elevated blood cholesterol levels. A thyroid imbalance must be carefully managed by a physician through blood tests and office evaluation so the proper dose can be described. Most people who suffer from thyroid conditions are female (90 percent of the total hypothyroid cases in the United States are women), so it is a common condition frequently seen by physicians who specialize in women's health care.

Whether you decide to use synthetic progestins, natural progesterone, or a low-dose birth control pill or other drug therapy, excessive bleeding problems can be controlled. You may need to try several dose regimens or forms of treatment if you encounter side effects. However, the decreased risk of excessive bleeding that these treatments provide is well worth the time spent finding a plan that is right for you.

12

Surgery for Relief of Irregular Menstruation

Many women with irregular and heavy menstrual bleeding never need surgery. Those with mild to moderate symptoms may handle the bleeding process quite effectively by practicing self-help methods or using drug and hormonal therapies. Remember that many of the problems that cause excessive bleeding are hormonally stimulated by estrogen and may become less severe with the onset of menopause when hormonal levels decrease. For example, fibroids and endometriosis are stimulated by high levels of estrogen. Conservative management may allow women to preserve their uterus and avoid the physical and emotional stress of surgery.

For some women, however surgery is unavoidable and necessary. In this chapter, I discuss the surgical techniques commonly used to treat these conditions as well as their indications and risks. Both conservative and more extensive surgical procedures can be performed to control the causes of bleeding. The conservative procedures include dilatation and curettage (D&C), endometrial dilation, myomectomy, and removal of implants for endometriosis. Extensive surgery includes hysterectomy and the more radical total abdominal hysterectomy

Conservative Surgical Procedures

Dilatation and Curettage

While dilatation and curettage is a very helpful procedure often used to diagnose the cause of bleeding, the D&C can also be therapeutic. Many physicians prefer the more easily performed endometrial biopsy to rule out hyperplasia or cancer as the cause of excessive bleeding. Occasionally doctors perform the more extensive diagnostic procedure called a D&C, particularly if the patient is experiencing heavy bleeding or polyps are suspected. The D&C requires anesthesia because the physician uses a scraping or suction technique to remove the lining of the uterus. Not only does this allow for the diagnosis of the problem through cell analysis, but the D&C also effectively stops the bleeding, at least temporarily.

Endometrial Ablation

This technique has been gaining prominence in recent years as a more conservative surgical approach to managing heavy bleeding. It involves the use of a laser or an electro-surgical technique to essentially render the lining of the uterus inactive. The procedure allows the uterus itself to remain intact while achieving a 97 percent success rate. Studies have shown that 50 percent of patients undergoing ablation cease menstruating entirely while the other 50 percent have slight spotting at the time of their menses following the procedure.

Myomectomy

This procedure solves the problem of heavy menstrual flow due to fibroid tumors. Younger women find this an important option because it removes the fibroid tumors while preserving the uterus, thus allowing for the possibility of childbearing. For those women whose infertility is caused by fibroids, up to 54 percent conceive following a myomectomy. Fibroids are responsible for up to ten percent of all cases of infertility. Also, the rate of spontaneous abortion due to fibroids drops substantially following myomectomy.

The surgeon may perform a myomectomy through a vaginal incision when the fibroids are located submucosally, or through an abdominal incision for intramural, subserosal, or pedunculated fibroids extending into the pelvis. Many surgeons will not perform a myomectomy when the uterine size becomes too enlarged or the patient has too many fibroids. Though the number and size of the fibroids are not an absolute technical deterrent in themselves, removal of a large number of these benign tumors may be beyond the scope of some surgeons. The number of fibroids that can be found once the uterus is exposed during surgery can be astonishing. Several dozen fibroids are not unusual and numbers as high as 200 have been reported. These can range from tiny seedling tumors to huge cysts weighing several pounds. If you want to consider a myomectomy, find a surgeon comfortable and very experienced with this technique.

A skilled surgeon can help minimize side effects from the procedure such as excessive blood loss from the surgery, as well as post-operative scarring or adhesions which can themselves impair fertility. Micro-surgical procedures that cause minimal tissue damage and control bleeding help minimize the development of inflammation and adhesions post-operatively. The use of laser technology instead of traditional surgical tools has been used more and more in recent years. Lasers do not change the basic surgical procedure, since the surgeon must still open up the patient and cut out the fibroids. However, surgeons skilled in the use of the lasers can do the procedure with significantly less bleeding. Some patients have reported less post-operative pain and more comfortable healing.

Myomectomy may not provide a definitive cure for fibroids. Follow-up studies, show a 15 to 45 percent risk of further growth of new tumors necessitating more surgery. The mortality rate for both procedures is nearly identical — on the order of one to two percent. For women who wish to preserve their uterus, myomectomy offers a viable option, if surgery must be performed.

Removal of Endometriosis Implants

Conservative surgery for endometriosis keeps the patient's reproductive organs intact while removing the endometriosis implants while the more extensive surgery removes both the implants and the reproductive organs. Normally, endometrial implants are diagnosed with a laparoscopy. The laparoscope is an instrument that allows visualization of the pelvic cavity and the reproductive organs. Once the implants, adhesions, endometrial cysts, or other changes typical of endometriosis are located, treatments can be initiated at once. In many cases, this prevents the need for a second, follow-up surgical procedure after diagnosis. Treatment consists of destroying the implants by the use of a laser or electrocautery. Either technique can remove scarring or adhesions, implants, and small ovarian cysts.

Some physicians prefer laser therapy because it decreases blood loss, reduces thermal damage to the tissues by the instrument, and lessens post-operative adhesions. Cautery should be avoided when treating the fallopian tubes or bladder because of the risk of burning these tissues. However, in the hands of an experienced surgeon, laser therapy and electrocautery techniques are extremely effective. To improve the cure rate, many physicians combine surgery with drug therapy like Danazol™. Medication is often given either pre- or postoperatively to further reduce the risk of recurrence.

There are women for whom laparoscopic surgery is not a good option. Women with severe endometriosis, numerous adhesions, involvement of the bowel or urinary tract, large endometrial cysts, or extensive disease in the ovaries may need more radical surgery. These problems are often beyond the scope of laser or cautery treatment and may require a larger incision and removal of the reproductive organs, as well as destruction of the implant and scar tissue.

How successful is conservative surgery? Not as successful as one would hope. Unfortunately, the recurrence rate after surgery is fairly high. One percent of patients have a recurrence of active endometriosis within the first year following surgery, while the three- and five-year recurrent rates are 13 and 40 percent, respectively. Some women will eventually require a second laparoscopic procedure or even a total abdominal hysterectomy as treatment for recurrence.

Extensive Surgical Procedures

These procedures not only remove the underlying pathological condition, but also the reproductive organs themselves. This can range from simple removal of the uterus to the removal of other pelvic structures such as the ovaries and fallopian tubes.

Hysterectomy

The presence of fibroids is one of the most common reasons for this procedure to be done in the United States. In fact, one-third of hyster-ectomies performed are done for fibroid treatment. In my opinion, some of these hysterectomies may not be necessary. Some doctors will suggest a hysterectomy if the uterus has become greatly enlarged, even in women with mild or no symptoms. In the absence of symptoms, size of the uterus alone is not a compelling reason for this operation. If the fibroid is not pressing on the bladder, rectum, or other pelvic structure, a woman may go for years without any resulting problems or discomfort at all. Eventually many of these tumors will shrink and even disappear with menopause.

Some women with very large asymptomatic fibroids may wish to have a hysterectomy for cosmetic reasons, if they cause significant protrusion or bulging of the abdominal wall. If your physician recommends a hysterectomy for fibroids that are symptom-free, I suggest that you get a second opinion from another physician in your area known to be more conservative in his or her management. In fact, a second opinion is always a good idea before undergoing any radical surgical procedure.

Strong indications for a hysterectomy include the following:

- Extremely heavy bleeding due to hormonal imbalance, premenopause, or fibroid tumors causing anemia or significant lifestyle problems.

- Attempts at conservative therapy that have been unsuccessful due to recurring fibroid tumors.

- Rapidly enlarging fibroid tumors with worsening pelvic pressure. In a post-menopausal woman, this requires careful evaluation because, on rare occasions, it may indicate a malignant process occurring in the uterus. (Fortunately, less than one-third of one percent of all fibroids are found to have malignant properties.)

- Fibroid tumors causing symptoms such as increased urinary frequency and constipation.

- A diagnosis of precancerous endometrial hyperplasia.

If you have any of these health issues or symptoms, a hysterectomy may be the correct and necessary therapy to treat the problem. For women who do not wish to preserve their fertility and childbearing capability, the decision to have a hysterectomy for one of these reasons may be a noncontroversial and definitive choice.

Before agreeing to have a hysterectomy, it is important that you be informed as to all the risks and benefits of the procedure. Patients must take responsibility for their bodies and learn as much as they can about the surgery. I consider good communication to be an essential part of a healthy doctor-patient relationship. Remember, this is one of the most important relationships that you will ever have in your life. Your physician plays an enormous role in helping to preserve your health and well-being, so be sure you feel comfortable with your doctor. Ask about the emotional and physical risks to you, how long recovery will take, and how you can expect to feel afterwards. Remember, your physician should have an enormous backlog of knowledge, because he or she has probably gone through this with thousands of other patients.

Complications may include blood loss significant enough to require a blood transfusion during surgery. Infections at the site of the incisions, or at other sites like the bladder or lung, may also occur post-operatively. All too often, women are simply not prepared for how they will feel after surgery.

I have had many patients who have consulted me after a hysterectomy. Although some women regain their strength and energy level rapidly, I have had patients who were shocked at how tired and depressed they felt for months after surgery. Though their surgeons had warned them that they should not lift heavy items and should avoid rigorous physical activity during the postoperative period, they received no warning that their quality of life might suffer, that they might feel more emotional and upset, or that their sexual enjoyment might diminish after removal of their uterus.

Many post hysterectomy patients looking to regain their pre-surgical zest and well-being have come to me for therapies based on lifestyle changes, such as an optimal nutritional program and stress management techniques. The self-help chapters of this book describe solutions I have found to be helpful for such patients.

Extensive Surgery for Endometriosis or Endometrial (Uterine) Cancer

Surgeons often recommend more extensive surgery in women in their thirties and forties who have more severe disease and in women for whom fertility is not an issue. A woman in her middle to late thirties or forties, in whom childbearing is completed or is not desired, may elect to undergo a more radical procedure in which the surgeon opens the abdomen and removes the uterus along with all visible implants and adhesions.

To avoid an early menopause, the surgeon should try to spare the ovaries if at all possible (or at least part of one ovary if the endometriosis has attached itself to these glands). In my practice, I have seen that a premature, surgically induced menopause can be difficult for women to tolerate when the ovaries are entirely removed. Symptoms like hot flashes and vaginal dryness can be quite severe. The risk of developing osteoporosis is greater in these women.

There is also a slight chance of reactivating the endometriosis in women who have had a total hysterectomy after they are placed on hormonal replacement therapy. This is because estrogen stimulates the growth of the implants. It may be impossible to remove every microscopic implant particle during the operation, thus leaving behind tissue such as the bladder and intestines that can reactivate and cause symptoms under hormonal stimulation. This can be a double-edge sword for younger women who don't want to suffer from hot flashes, yet are concerned about possible hormonal side effects.

Therefore, I strongly believe in preserving ovarian function if at all possible in women who must undergo surgery for endometriosis. Unfortunately, complete removal of the ovaries, fallopian tubes, and uterus is common, particularly for women in their forties and even when the disease is entirely treatable by removal of only the implants and scar tissue.

Endometrial cancer tends to occur in an older population than endometriosis. The maximum incidence is in the two decades between 50 and 70 years. Thus, endometrial cancer tends to be a problem seen primarily in postmenopausal women. Even with early stage cancer, the treatment usually involves a total hysterectomy with removal of both ovaries and fallopian tubes. If the tumor is diagnosed in an advanced stage, meaning that it has spread to sites outside the uterus such as the liver, lungs, or upper abdomen, progestins (synthetic progesterone) and chemotherapy may also be utilized as part of the treatment program. Radiation therapy may also be given to certain patients in an attempt to prevent the disease from recurring.

If either a hysterectomy or a hysterectomy with removal of the fallopian tubes and uterus is determined to be necessary, I recommend that patients choose their surgeon carefully, with the goal of preserving as many of their reproductive organs as possible without sacrificing the best therapeutic response. If major surgery is required, it is important to speak with several doctors to learn what options are available.

13

How to Put Your Program Together

This book provides a complete self-help program to prevent and relieve your symptoms. The Complete Treatment Chart summarizes the many treatment options presented in this book. Use this chart for reference as you devise your own program. Try the treatment options that feel most comfortable to you. You may find, for example, in trying the exercises or the stress-reduction techniques, that certain routines feel better to you than others. If that is the case, practice those that bring the greatest sense of relief for your particular symptoms.

Always keep in mind that your ultimate goal is relief of your irregular and heavy menstrual bleeding problem resulting in a major improvement in your overall health and well-being. I generally recommend beginning any self-help program slowly so that you have the time to get comfortable with the lifestyle changes. Everyone has a different capacity for adjusting to major changes in lifestyle. While some of my patients like to eliminate their old, unhealthy habits as quickly as possible, many other women find such rapid changes in their long-term habits to be too stressful. Find the pace that works for you.

Enjoy the program. I always tell my patients to regard their self-help program as an enjoyable adventure. The exercises and stress reduction techniques should give you a sense of energy and well-being. The menus and food selections in this book provide you with an opportunity to try delicious and healthful new foods.

As you do the program, don't set unrealistic or too strict expectations for yourself. You don't have to be perfect to get great results. Just follow the guidelines of the program as well as you can and as your schedule permits.

It is not a disaster if you forget to take your vitamins occasionally or don't have time to exercise on any particular day. Don't be discouraged if you can't follow the dietary recommendations on vacations, holidays, and birthdays. Periodically, review the guidelines outlined in this book and continue to adapt your lifestyle to the healthful suggestions that I've shared with you. Over time you will notice many beneficial changes.

Be your own feedback system. Your body will tell you if you are on the right track and if what you are doing is making you feel better. It will also tell you if your diet and emotional stresses are increasing your symptoms. Remember that even moderate changes in your habits can make significant differences.

The Irregular Menstruation Workbook

At the start of your program, fill out the workbook section of this book. The workbook questionnaires will help you evaluate which areas in your life have contributed most to your symptoms and need the most work. Use the workbook every month or two as you follow the self-help program. The workbook will help you see the areas in which you are making the most progress, both with symptom relief and with the initiation of healthier lifestyle habits. The workbook can give you organized and easy-to-use feedback on your progress with the program.

Diet and Nutritional Supplements

I recommend that you make all nutritional changes gradually. Many women find breakfast the easiest meal to change because it is simple and often eaten at home. To change your other meals and snacks, periodically review the list of foods to avoid and foods to emphasize. Each month pick a few foods that you are willing to eliminate from your diet. Try the foods that help prevent and relieve irregular and heavy menstrual bleeding. The recipes and menus included in this book should be very helpful as you restructure your diet.

Vitamins, minerals, and herbal supplements can help complete your nutritional needs and speed up the healing process. They are a very important part of the program for most women.

Stress Reduction

The stress-reduction exercises play an important role in facilitating the physical healing process. I find that all my patients heal more rapidly from almost any problem when they are calm, happy, and relaxed. The visualization exercises actually help you set a blue-print in your mind for optimal health. This allows the body and mind to work together in harmony.

Begin the program initially by putting aside 15 to 30 minutes each day, depending on the flexibility of your schedule. Try all the stress-reduction exercises listed in this book. Choose the combination that works best for you. Practice stress management on a regular basis.

You do not need to spend enormous amounts of time on these exercises. Many women are too busy to spend an hour a day meditating. Even 10 minutes out of your daily schedule can be helpful. You may find that the quietest times for you are early in the morning before you get out of bed or late at night before going to sleep. Other women simply choose to take a break during the day. You can close the door to your office or go into your bedroom at home for 10 minutes to relax. Use the time to breathe deeply, do the visualizations, or meditate. You will be much calmer and more relaxed afterward.

Exercise

You should exercise on a regular basis, at least three times a week. Women with heavy menstrual bleeding may find that vigorous exercise is too stressful and tiring. Follow the gentle stretches and acupressure exercises in this book. Aerobic exercise such as walking should be done slowly and comfortably and never to the point of exhaustion. It is important that women who are tired, because of heavy menstrual bleeding, keep their muscles and joints flexible and supple. This will help combat fatigue by enhancing circulation to all parts of the body. Try the fitness and flexibility exercises in this book.

To do the stretches and acupressure exercises described in this book, set aside a half-hour each day for the first week or two of your self-help program. Try all the exercises. After an initial period of exploration, choose the ones that you enjoy most and that seem to give you the most relief. Practice them on a regular basis so that they can help prevent and reduce your symptoms.

Conclusion

I wish to reaffirm that each of us can do a tremendous amount for ourselves to assure optimal health and well-being. By having access to information, education, and health resources, every woman can play a major role in creating her own state of good health. Practice the beneficial self-help techniques outlined in this book. Follow good nutritional habits, exercise, and practice regular stress-reduction techniques.

By combining good principles of self-care along with your regular medical care, you can enjoy the same wonderful results that my patients and I have had for a life of good health and well-being.

About Susan Richards, M.D.

Dr. Susan Richards is one of the foremost authorities in the fields of family medicine and alternative medicine. Dr. Richards has successfully treated many thousands of patients emphasizing alternative health and integrative medicine in her clinical practice. Her mission is to provide her patients with safe and effective alternative therapies to greatly enhance their health and well-being.

A graduate of Northwestern University Feinberg School of Medicine, she has served on the clinical faculty of Stanford University School of Medicine and taught in their Division of Family and Community Medicine.

Her Facebook page, Dr. Susan's Healthy Living, has over one million followers. She is also an ordained minister and her ministry receives over a million prayer requests for healing each year.

Notes

Notes

References

Am 3 J Obstet Gynecol. 1977 Mar 15;127(6):572-80.;

Am J Clin Nutr. 2007 Jun;85(6):1586-91.}

Am J Epidemiol. 2009 Jul 1;170(1):12-23.

Baber R, Bligh PC, Fulcher G, et al. The effect of an Isoflavone dietary supplement (P-081) on serum lipids, forearm bone density & endometrial thickness in post menopausal women [abstract]. Menopause. 1999a;6:326. Baber RJ, Templeman C, Morton T, et al. Randomized, placebo-controlled trial of an isoflavone supplement and menopausal symptoms in women. Climacteri

Carcinogenesis. 2008 Jan;29(1):93-9.

Cassady 3M, Zennie TM, Young-Heum C, et al. Use of a mammalian cell culture benzo(a)pyrene metabolism assay for the detection of potential anticarcinog(from natural products: Inhibition of metabolism by biochanin A, anisoflavone from Trifolium pratense L. Cancer Res. 1988;48:6257-6261.

Chedraui P, San Miguel G, Hidalgo L, Morocho N, Ross S. Effect of Trifolium pratense-derived isoflavones on the lipid profile of postmenopausal women with increased body mass index. Gynecol Endocrinol. 2008 Nov;24(11):620-4.

DerMarderosian A, ed. Red Clover. In: Facts and Comparisons The Review of Natural Products. 5th ed. Philadelphia, Pa: Lippincott Williams & Wilkins; 2008 Duke JA. CRC Handbook of Medicinal Herbs. Boca Raton, Fla: CRC Press, Inc.; 2000:614.

Engl J Med. 1975 Dec 4;293(23):1167-70.;

Fertil Steril. 2003 Jan;79(1):221-2.

Geller SE, Studee L. Soy and red clover for mid-life and aging. Climacteric. 2006 Aug;9(4):245-63.

Heck AM, DeWitt BA, Lukes AL. Potential interactions between alternative therapies and warfarin. Am 1 Health Syst Pharm. 2000;57(13):1221-1227.

Howes 3B, Sullivan D, Lai N. The effects of dietary supplementation with isoflavones from red clover on the lipoprotein profiles of postmenopausal women w mild to moderate hypercholesterolemia. Atherosclerosis. 2000;152(1):143-147.

Husband A. Red clover isoflavone supplements: safety and pharmacokinetics. Journal of the British Menopause Society. 2001;Supplement S1:4-7.

J Steroid Biochem Mol Biol. 2007 Mar;103(3-5):708-11.

Jeri AR. The effect of isoflavones phytoestrogens in relieving hot flushes in Peruvian postmenopausal women. Paper presented at: 9th International Menopai Society World Congress on the Menopause; October 20, 1999; Yokahama, Japan.

Kuhn MA, Winston D. Herbal Therapy and Supplements. Philadelphia, Pa: Lippincott; 2008:365-369

Lancet. 1999 May 29;353(9167):1824-8.1999b; 2(2): 85-92.

McGuffin M, Hobbs C, Upton R, et al. Botanical Safety Handbook. Boca Raton, Fla: CRC Press LLC; 1997: 117.

Mueller M, Jungbauer A. Red clover extract: a putative source for simultaneous treatment of menopausal disorders and the metabolic syndrome. Menopause 2008 Nov-Dec; 15(6): 1120-31.

Nachtigall LE. Isoflavones in the management of menopause. Journal of the British Menopause Society. 2001;Supplement S1:8-12.

Nestel P3, Pomeroy S, Kay S, et al. Isoflavones from red clover improve systemic arterial compliance but not plasma lipids in menopausal women. J din Endocrinol Metab. 1999;84(3):895-898.

North American Menopause Society (NAMS). The role of isoflavones in menopausal health: consensus opinion of the North American Menopause Society. Menopause. 2000;7(4):215-229.

Occhiuto F, Pasquale RD, Guglielmo G, Palumbo DR, Zangla G, Samperi S, Renzo A, Circosta C. Effects of phytoestrogenic isoflavones from red clover (Trifoli pratense L.) on experimental osteoporosis. Phytother Res. 2007 Feb;21(2):130-4.

Powles TJ, Howell A, Evans DG, McCloskey EV, Ashley S, Greenhalgh R, Affen 3, Flook LA, Tidy A. Red clover isoflavones are safe and well tolerated in women with a family history of breast cancer. Menopause Int. 2008 Mar;14(1):6-12.

Rakel: Integrative Medicine, 2nd ed. Philadelphia, PA: Saunders Elsevier, Inc. 2007.

Stephens FO. Phytoestrogens and prostate cancer: possible preventive role. MJA. 1997;167:138-140.

Tang NP, Li H, Qiu YL, Zhou GM, Ma J. Am J Obstet Gynecol. 2009 Dec;201(6):605.e1-8. Epub 2009 Sep 20. PMID: 19766982 [PubMed - indexed for MEDLINE]

Umland EM. Treatment strategies for reducing the burden of menopause-associated vasomotor symptoms. J Manag Care Pharm. 2008 Apr;14(3 Suppl):14-S Review.

Voskuil DW, Monninkhof EM, Elias SG, Vlems FA, van Leeuwen FE; Task Force Physical Activity and Cancer. Cancer Epidemiol Biomarkers Prey. 2007 Apr;16(4):639-48. Review. PMID: 17416752 [PubMed - indexed for MEDLINE] Free Article.

Woodside 3V, Campbell MI Isoflavones and breast cancer. Journal of the British Menopause Society. 2001;Supplement S1:17-21.

Wuttke W, Rimoldi G, Christoffel 3, Seidlova-Wuttke D. Plant extracts for the treatment of menopausal women: Safe? Maturitas. 2006 Nov 1;55 Suppl 1:S92 S100. Epub 2006 Aug 8.

Zava DT, Dollbaum CM, Blen M. Estrogen and progestin bioactivity of foods, herbs, and spices. Proc Soc Exp Biol Med. 1998;217(3):369-378.